My Family and Food Allergies

The All You Need to Know Guide

ALEXA BARACAIA

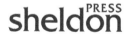

First published in Great Britain by Sheldon Press in 2021
An imprint of John Murray Press
A division of Hodder & Stoughton Ltd,
An Hachette UK company

1

Copyright © Alexa Baracaia 2021

A CIP catalogue record for this title is available from the British Library

Trade Paperback ISBN 9781529349887
eBook ISBN 9781529349894

Typeset by KnowledgeWorks Global Ltd.

Printed and bound in Great Britain by Clays Ltd, Elcograf S.p.A.

John Murray Press policy is to use papers that are natural, renewable and
recyclable products and made from wood grown in sustainable forests.
The logging and manufacturing processes are expected to conform to the
environmental regulations of the country of origin.

John Murray Press
Carmelite House
50 Victoria Embankment
London EC4Y 0DZ

Nicholas Brealey Publishing
Hachette Book Group
Market Place, Center 53, State Street
Boston, MA 02109, USA

www.sheldonpress.co.uk

For Sidney, the inspiration and driving force behind this book, and Sadie, who loves an 'eggy pancake' but is always looking out for her big brother.

Contents

Contributors

With heartfelt thanks and gratitude to the army of amazing allergy specialists who helped and guided me in the writing of this book.

First and foremost, to our own allergy consultant Dr Robert Boyle, who has provided his time, wisdom, support and unending patience in clinically reviewing much of the medical detail contained here. Also, huge thanks for everything over the years since diagnosis. It has been a privilege to have 'Dr Bob' on hand as a calm, positive and reassuring presence, always ready to answer our questions and allay our fears. I know we have struck it lucky. May every allergy family be blessed with a Dr Bob!

Thank you to Dr Mary Halsey, whose significant contribution and expertise informs the very important chapters on managing anxiety, as well as other elements woven in throughout this book. On the same topic, my great thanks to Dr Kate Roberts and Dr Rebecca Knibb.

Thank you to Dr Lauri-Ann van der Poel, for so generously and methodically going through my chapter on eczema, hay fever and asthma, and offering both hard-pressed time and support.

Thanks to Carina Venter, for answering my frantic questions over opposing time zones, and sharing her considerable knowledge; to Professor George du Toit for support and guidance on food challenges, immunotherapy and more; to Dr Mich Lajeunesse for making himself available for video interview on immunotherapy and hopes for the future; and to Dr Paul Turner for sharing invaluable papers and guidance.

Thank you also to the formidable triumvirate of Dr Hazel Gowland, Adrian Rogers and Alex Gazzola for sharing considerable expertise over so many messages, calls and emails, and patiently helping me to navigate the tricky topics of food and cosmetics labelling, 'may contain' warnings and very much more.

More thanks are due to Tracey Dunn, to Marisha Cysewski and Joanna Abishegam-David of the Food Standards Agency, and to Dr Paul Seddon, Dr Tariq El-Shanawany and Dr Adrian Sie.

So many experts have so generously helped me that I'm scared I may inadvertently miss someone out. But I am truly grateful to all, and this book would have remained a puddle of unformed panic without you. Thank you.

Acknowledgements

These very special thanks are for the other army – my fellow allergy parents, friends and family whose care, counsel, understanding and wisdom form the backbone (and heart) of this book. Your experience and support are everything.

Namechecking everyone would be an impossible feat, but to all those who offered up their stories, and to everyone I have met and connected with and spent hours chatting to on Twitter, and during #allergyhour – thank you. Thank you for being there, and for sharing, supporting, laughing, raging and campaigning. Special thanks among these to Kate and family in the Barcelona sunshine, the Kick Ass Mamas, and Clare H.

Thanks to Bev Dickinson and Heather Corbett, who have been amazing and wonderful looking after S and his allergy/med needs at school. Sending never-ending Pimm's to Bev for always answering my emails with cheer and speed – it's honestly meant the world.

The biggest thank you to family: to Nanny, Nonno, Aunty Simi, Uncle Dan, Elliott, Cassia, Grandma and Grandad for always making sure S is included: cellophaning the mayonnaise; creating a 'Sidney-safe' cupboard; adapting birthday cakes; for flapjacks, Christmas gingerbread people, homemade ice cream and holidays. Oh – and for always checking the labels!

To friends who have taken on caring for or catering for S, I can't tell you how much it's appreciated. Thank you for every Pizza Express or Nando's kids' party, every pack of safe popcorn brought in for a class birthday, every 'is this biscuit OK?', every Haribo in a party bag. These little things mean more than you will ever know.

Thank you to Lucy Finnemore of Higher Lank Farm in glorious Cornwall, the first person outside of our family that we ever trusted to cook for Sidney, whose allergy-friendly High Tea remains the stuff of legend, and to whom we return year after year.

And lastly, but most importantly, to my Lego-loving Sidney, who is always happiest when well-fed, and remains largely unbothered by this big fuss about allergies. To his little sister Sadie, my bundle of chatter and song, who loves and looks out for her big brother always (even when they're fighting).

And to my lovely husband and team-mate Paul, for stopping me from rifling through bins to check labels, backing me up all the way, taking on interminable hours of lockdown home-schooling and duck-feeding so I could write this book, and of course being the best dad Sidney and Sadie could ever have.

Introduction

Scrambled eggs on Mother's Day

It was Mother's Day breakfast that booted us into a new way of life. And the morning had started so well: just a couple of night-time wake-ups and a respectable 7 a.m. start from our five-month-old baby boy. Flowers (pink and yellow) delivered to the door. Cards. A cup of tea in bed. And scrambled eggs on toast.

Then, not long after, we noticed an odd rash developing on his legs: white, bumpy, like nettle stings. Within minutes the lumps had spread to his throat and chin. He was by now red in the face, crying loudly, obviously in some distress.

My husband recognized hives: he carries an EpiPen for a ridiculous list of food sensitivities that transform him into the Elephant Man when combined with vigorous exercise (that's one for another book). We got on the phone to my sister, a doctor. She said: 'Call an ambulance.'

So, the rest of my first Mother's Day was spent, memorably enough, languishing in a Hackney A&E. A syringe full of antihistamine saw off the lumps and bumps but we were baffled as to what had caused this reaction when he was still solely breastfed. Was it the flowers? Pollen in the early spring air? Something in his eczema creams (we'd been battling skin rashes since he was just a few weeks old)? The paediatric team couldn't say – just go straight back to the GP or A&E if it happens again.

Barely a month later it did, and this time the cause was blindingly obvious. I gave him his first taste of banana. Within minutes there were red splodges where the mash had touched his skin, and soon hives had spread across his face and neck.

Another dash to the doctor and a request, now, for specialist referral.

We were due to go on holiday with my parents just a couple of weeks later, and the wait to see an allergy specialist on the NHS would be at least three months, we were told. 'Try not to give him any new foods for now,' added the GP. Other than banana, his diet had reached the giddy heights of baby rice, sweet potato and broccoli. It didn't seem much for the next three months.

Panicked as to what might have caused it, and worried about whether the next reaction would be more serious, we booked to see an NHS consultant privately. He asked us to run through exactly what had happened on the morning of the first reaction. We blathered about pollen and flowers, skin creams, floor cleaners. He asked what we had eaten. Scrambled eggs, we said. 'That'll be it,' he said. He hadn't even eaten any, we protested, stupidly. But the results of a skin prick test confirmed it: our baby was allergic to egg. Apparently even a trace on our hands, unwittingly transferred to his poor broken skin when we were applying his creams, would have been enough to trigger the hives.

Of course, we weren't surprised when banana threw up a positive (though who had ever heard of banana allergy?). Possibly wheat, too, though the results were borderline. Plus sesame. And peanuts.

The rest is a long and boring story, but the upshot is this: we were sent home clutching a bottle of antihistamines, a prescription for two EpiPens, three pamphlets on nut-free, wheat-free and egg-free diets, a good deal of sensible advice from the doctor and dietitian and now, ten and a half years on, here we are.

We've added and removed a few on the list since then: he soon developed pea, chickpea and red lentil allergies, which he later outgrew. Allergies like to keep you on your toes. Various tree nuts were a problem early on, but he has since been able to include them safely in his diet. Banana and wheat resolved, but we're left with peanuts, egg and sesame today. I won't bore you with the Oral Allergy Syndrome (more on that later) that generously decided to develop during the first coronavirus lockdown, but raw hazelnuts, raw carrots and nectarines are now off the menu, too.

It's been something of a rollercoaster, that's for sure. I've learned a few things along the way. Allergy isn't straightforward. No two people are the same; no two reactions are the same. Some allergies you will outgrow; others you will not. Some new ones will pop up; others you will navigate brilliantly.

It's also surprising how quickly you get used to this weird new way of life, where food – previously a benign source of comfort and nourishment – becomes a threat and a source of intense anxiety. Often, it's having to explain the complexities of what we can and can't have to other people that's the problem.

The biggest thing, really, is trying to keep him safe from harm, bring him up aware but unafraid, and all while never, ever wanting him to feel like the funny allergic kid.

1

How to explain food allergy to others (and remind yourself)

Simply put, an allergy is an abnormally high sensitivity to a certain substance, such as a food, pollen or drugs. Food allergy is also sometimes termed 'food hypersensitivity'.

The word 'allergy' is derived from the Greek 'allos', meaning different or strange, and 'ergon', meaning activity. Allergies can range from the irritating runny nose and itchy eyes you get during hay fever season to potentially life-threatening reactions.

One huge frustration for families dealing with severe or chronic allergies is how easily the term is bandied about with little understanding. A common cause for confusion is when the words 'allergy' and 'intolerance' are used interchangeably. Hopefully this guide should help you unpick the vocab.

Food intolerance

The key thing to know about a food intolerance is that, unlike a food allergy, it does not involve the immune system. Symptoms typically occur slowly, after eating significant amounts of a particular food, and usually because the body has trouble processing that food effectively. Because there is often no diagnostic test for food intolerance, and because symptoms can be varied and may present longer after eating than with food allergy, they can take time to diagnose.

While symptoms are not as potentially dangerous as food allergy reactions, they can be debilitating and distressing. Symptoms include bloating, diarrhoea, nausea or vomiting. Other signs include fatigue, eczema or joint pains.

Many food intolerances involve the digestive system. For example, lactose intolerance is a condition where the body can't digest lactose, a sugar found in cow's milk. Foods high in histamine, such as wine and cheese, can also be culprits, while wheat intolerance – or wheat sensitivity – may be an issue for some.

Food allergy

Our immune system works by protecting us from invading organisms that can cause illness. If you have an allergy, your immune system mistakes an otherwise harmless substance as an invader. This substance, usually a small protein within a certain food, is called an 'allergen'.

What most of us understand to be food allergy is known as **IgE-mediated food allergy**, in which the immune system overreacts to the allergen by producing Immunoglobulin E (IgE) antibodies. These travel to cells that release histamine and other chemicals, causing an allergic reaction.[1]

Symptoms of food allergy usually occur within 30 minutes of eating and may involve tingling or itching in the lips, tongue, mouth or throat. There may also be runny or itchy eyes and sneezing, as well as abdominal pain, nausea or vomiting, swelling of the lips, face or eyes (known as 'angioedema') and sometimes – not always – a nettle-type rash known as hives or urticaria. Other rare and more serious symptoms may include swelling of the throat, difficulty breathing, wheezing, chest tightness or breathlessness – termed 'anaphylaxis' or an 'anaphylactic reaction'.

Just to complicate things a little further, there is another type of food allergy that also involves the immune system (making it distinct from an 'intolerance') but that isn't caused by IgE

---

1 British Society for Allergy & Clinical Immunology. See: <https://www.bsaci.org/patients/frequently-asked-questions/>

antibodies. This is known as **non-IgE-mediated food allergy**. These sorts of reactions are caused by other cells in the immune system and can take up to several hours – even two days – to develop. As a result, this type of allergy is harder to diagnose. Symptoms can occur over a longer period, such as eczema, diarrhoea, constipation and, in more severe cases, growth problems.

People can have either IgE-mediated or non-IgE-mediated food allergies, and some may experience symptoms from both types. Remember, too, that allergies are not one size fits all. A reaction can cause different symptoms in different people and even different symptoms in the same person each time it occurs: an egg allergy, say, can cause an itchy rash on one occasion and vomiting on the next.

To complicate things further still (gah, that's the thing about food allergies!), symptoms of an allergic reaction may be the same as the symptoms of some non-allergic conditions. For example, hives or swelling are **not** always due to allergies – they may, for instance, be caused by viral or bacterial infections or side effects from some medicines – so proper diagnosis of their cause is vital to get the right treatment.

People with an intolerance can usually eat small amounts of the food to which they are intolerant. In contrast, allergic reactions to foods usually occur quickly and can be life-threatening. People with allergies to foods usually react to small amounts of the food.

'The distinction between allergies and intolerance is important because it changes the advice given. Unfortunately, food allergies and intolerances are often confused, which can result in risky behaviour if you have a severe allergy, and needlessly strict avoidance if you have an intolerance.' – Dr Tariq El-Shanawany, Consultant Clinical Immunologist [2]

---

2 'Sense About Science: Making Sense of Allergies'. See: <https://archive. senseaboutscience.org/data/files/resources/189/Making-Sense-of-Allergies.pdf>

What's atopy?

This is a word you'll probably hear a fair bit. If someone is 'atopic' it means they are genetically predisposed to allergic disease. This may include hay fever, asthma, eczema and food allergy. It tends to run in families, although having a parent with a food allergy, or asthma, for instance, doesn't mean a child will automatically also go on to develop these conditions.

However, an Isle of Wight study[3] found atopic disease to be more common in children with one or more atopic parent, and that a family history of atopy was the 'single most important risk factor for atopy in the children'.

Other food-related reactions

Oral Allergy Syndrome (OAS)

This is related to pollen, usually birch pollen, and is also sometimes known as 'Pollen Food Syndrome'.

A person who suffers from OAS will experience immediate allergic symptoms in the lips, mouth and throat when they eat certain raw fruits, vegetables and/or nuts. Most commonly these will take the form of itching or tingling, although there may be some swelling. There may also be redness, tummy pain, sneezing, or runny eyes or nose. Most people with OAS will only experience mild to moderate symptoms and it is rare to experience more serious reactions.

It can, however, be difficult to differentiate between the symptoms of OAS and food allergy, so it is important to seek medical advice for confirmation of any diagnosis.

---

3 'The prevalence of and risk factors for atopy in early childhood: a whole population birth cohort study', Tariq et al, *The Journal of Allergy & Clinical Immunology*, 1998. See: <https://www.jacionline.org/article/S0091-6749(98)70164-2/fulltext>

In children this syndrome can develop over time, often in later primary or teenage years. It is frequently preceded by the development of hay fever symptoms, and that's because OAS is a 'cross reactive' condition. The person is usually allergic to one or more pollen, whose proteins are similar to those in certain raw fresh fruit, vegetables and nuts. The immune system mistakes the food for pollen, sparking a reaction – even in food they have eaten without a hitch all their life.

In the UK, the biggest culprit is silver birch pollen, which tends to cause symptoms between March and May. Sometimes grass pollen can trigger OAS – or both together.

The most common foods affecting those with OAS are raw fruits (for example, apples, apricots, pears, cherries, kiwi, mango, plums, peaches, nectarines and tomatoes) and raw vegetables (for example, carrots and celery). A number of other plant foods may occasionally cause the condition, including raw or stir-fried legumes, such as mangetout, beansprouts and raw peas. The nuts usually involved in pollen food syndrome are hazelnut, almond and walnut.

If you experience an itchy mouth after eating the same type of food, make sure you see your GP or allergy specialist. With OAS you should avoid the raw food. Often these same foods can be tolerated when cooked or processed: cooked carrot or apple; peach yoghurts; tinned fruit and roasted hazelnuts may all provoke no symptoms.

An OAS reaction can be eased by washing your mouth out and with a dose of antihistamine. Be cautious when trying new foods and begin with small amounts.

Our story

Allergies have the uncanny knack of striking when you least expect them. We were trundling uneventfully along during the first lockdown of 2020 – as many of us remarked at the time, being an allergy parent is an awful lot like living in a pandemic. Washing hands, cleaning surfaces, staying vigilant, avoiding the thing that might make you ill, feeling like you're missing out on fun stuff ... and realising that life is a balance of carefully judged risks.

Things were actually easier on the allergy front: no need to cart the EpiPen to school and back or deal with unexpected parties or trips away. No restaurant meals to navigate, or family gatherings.

We were eating a perfectly normal lunch on a spring day in the garden; one we'd had many times before – wraps with carrot salad – when my son started coming out in blotches and complaining of an itchy tongue. Obviously, I panicked – had I given him wraps with a 'may contain sesame' warning? Had a bird dropped a peanut out of the sky and on to his plate? (Half joking – it did cross my mind.) We whisked his food away, poor kid, and gave him antihistamine.

Then, the next time we had carrot the same thing happened. He'd developed hay fever symptoms the year before: sneezing and snuffling in the park. His doctor confirmed it sounded like OAS.

A few weeks later, driving along a remote country lane somewhere around the back of Devon (but of course, where else would a new allergy choose to strike?), I handed over a pot of chopped nectarine for the kids to snack on, when he said his throat felt itchy and 'like it has a lump in it'. I doled out the antihistamine with shaky hands, and we diverted to the nearest hospital car park – thankfully close by – until the symptoms died away. His allergist confirmed OAS again: nectarines are another common culprit. Raw hazelnuts were also added to the list, and now we're just hoping we can keep it at that. I think it's a case of 'watch this space'.

Latex Food Syndrome

There is another 'cross reactive' syndrome that affects some people who are allergic to latex. It's less common than OAS, and more likely to occur in people who come into regular contact with latex, such as healthcare workers or those that have undergone multiple surgical procedures. The foods implicated include avocado, banana, kiwi and chestnut, and symptoms are often similar to those described for pollen-related reactions.

FPIES (Food Protein-Induced Enterocolitis Syndrome)

FPIES is a type of food allergy that affects the gastrointestinal tract, and mainly affects infants – somewhere around one in 300. Classic symptoms are repeated vomiting within two to four hours of trying a new food, sometimes with diarrhoea and dehydration, causing lethargy and change in body temperature and blood pressure.

Symptoms may not be as immediate as IgE food allergies, and, unlike IgE food allergies, they will not show up on standard allergy tests. In infants, FPIES reactions are most often caused by cow's milk protein and grains such as rice and oats. In older children and adults the condition is rare, but can be triggered by fish or shellfish.

A diagnosis would need to be made by a doctor examining the patient's history. Management is fairly straightforward: avoid the food, and the condition usually resolves in time, typically by around the age of three. Specialist input from a dietitian or doctor is advised to supervise reintroduction of the food, however. Visit <fpiesuk.org> for more information.

Coeliac disease

Coeliac disease is commonly described as an autoimmune disease where the body attacks its own cells, although most immunologists and allergists would argue that it is a non-IgE mediated allergy to gluten – this is because there are no symptoms in the absence of the trigger (gluten).

Eating gluten, a protein in wheat, rye and barley, causes the body to destroy and damage the lining of the small intestine and can sometimes cause symptoms in other parts of the body. Common symptoms include bloating, diarrhoea, nausea, constipation, tiredness and weight loss. Visit <coeliac.org.uk> for more information.

EoE (Eosinophilic Oesophagitis)

Less common than these other conditions is eosinophilic (pronounced ee-oh-sin-oh-fil-ik) oesophagitis, which affects around one in 10,000 people. Often misdiagnosed because symptoms can mimic more common diseases, they affect the gut and are identified by the elevated presence of a type of inflammatory white blood cell called an eosinophil. They are often found in those with a family history of allergic diseases such as hay fever, asthma or eczema. The body wants to attack a substance – for example, an allergy-triggering food – and releases a variety of toxins.

Symptoms depend on age but are usually related to difficulty in getting food down the oesophagus (the tube going from mouth to stomach). Food might feel like it's travelling down slowly or getting stuck.

People with EoE may experience stomach pain after eating, and vomiting. The causes are not fully understood but certain foods can trigger EoE, including mainly milk, egg, wheat and soy. It is a chronic disorder that needs a referral to an EoE expert allergist and gastroenterologist for diagnosis and management. Visit <gutscharity.org.uk> for more information.

Common causes of allergy

A number of different allergens are responsible for allergic reactions – from pollen to dust, food, insect stings, animal dander, mould, medication and latex.

Up to one in 12 children suffer from a food allergy, with the most frequent including:

- Egg
- Peanuts and tree nuts
- Milk
- Seeds
- Fish.

Cow's milk allergy

One of the more common allergies among children, milk allergy will usually become apparent in infancy. It may also be known as Cow's Milk Protein Allergy, or CMPA. More often than not it is outgrown in early childhood, on average by the age of five.

Children may have an immediate IgE-mediated allergy – with symptoms including rash, swelling, itching and difficulty breathing. Or, they may have a delayed non-IgE allergy, occurring between two to 72 hours after consumption and where symptoms include abdominal cramps, diarrhoea or frequent discoloured or frothy stools with mucus streaks of blood. Some children suffer from a mix of the two. Delayed onset non-IgE allergy is often outgrown sooner than IgE-mediated allergy to milk.

It can be very hard to differentiate between non-IgE milk allergy and other common childhood conditions, such as eczema, reflux, colic or constipation. Indeed, there have been concerns in recent years about the possible 'overdiagnosis' of cow's milk allergy, with perfectly normal symptoms potentially being over-interpreted.

A useful clue is the milk a child is being fed. Babies on formula milk who have severe symptoms of colic or reflux might have CMPA, but this is very unlikely in a breastfed baby, since they are not being fed milk protein other than minute quantities from the mother's diet. Only around 0.5 per cent of infants (one in 200) react to the cow's milk protein found in maternal breastmilk.

The British Society for Allergy & Clinical Immunology (BSACI) has produced guidance on the diagnosis of milk allergy, available via its website <https://www.bsaci.org/wp-content/uploads/2021/01/Summary-of-BSACI-Milk-Allergy-Guidelines-for-PC-FINAL-.pdf>.

There are no tests for delayed allergy, so these infants will require a supervised elimination diet under the care of a doctor or dietitian.

If you suspect CMPA, please visit your GP to discuss your concerns. It may be helpful to keep a diary of symptoms to take to your doctor:

- What are they?
- How old was your child when they first developed?
- How quickly do they develop after feeding?
- How often do they happen?

Consider taking photographs or videos of your infant feeding and of their skin, if and when it flares up.

If you decide to go dairy free while breastfeeding, you probably don't need to avoid dairy in baked foods. Ask a dietitian for advice to ensure you are getting enough calcium. If you are formula feeding, you may be recommended a hypoallergenic infant formula – available on prescription. Lactose-free milk is **not** suitable as it still contains the milk proteins that cause allergic reactions.

Hypoallergenic formulas contain cow's milk proteins that have been 'extensively hydrolysed' or broken down. These are well tolerated by infants with CMPA but are not usually needed after the age of one.

Those with more severe symptoms, or who cannot tolerate hypoallergenic formula, may be prescribed an amino acid formula, which does not contain cow's milk proteins. These infants should be referred to their local paediatric allergy service for proper assessment. Amino acid formula is also not usually needed after the age of one.

Soy milks are not suitable before the age of six months, and rice milks are not advised before the age of four and a half, but other plant-based milks such as oat, almond or coconut may be appropriate cow's milk substitutes for your child after the age of one. Your dietitian should advise you on which milk substitutes are suitable, but they should be fortified with calcium wherever possible.

Milks from other mammals – goats, for example – are not recommended as they share similar proteins to cow's milk. There is some suggestion that donkey and camel milk are less likely to cause symptoms but you should discuss this with your specialist first (also, I can't vouch for the palatability of camel milk on cornflakes!).

Young children with cow's milk allergy may be advised to carry out a hospital supervised baked milk 'challenge' (see Chapter 3) to see if they can tolerate this. There is no 'hard and fast rule' as to what age this may take place, although it is generally over the age of one.

For children with non-IgE milk allergy, there is a plan called the 'milk ladder' that progresses through various steps to, eventually, milk in its non-baked form. This should only be attempted under medical guidance.

Milk has to be declared as an ingredient in food, but watch out for less obvious sources such as breads and pastries, pasta, sauces, desserts, sweets and chocolates, lemon curd, chocolate spreads, ready meals, hot chocolate, soups, salad creams and mayo. Check every label.

An elimination diet to diagnose cow's milk allergy should be carried out under the guidance of a GP, a registered dietitian or an allergy clinic. It involves removing cow's milk from a child's diet for two to four weeks and then reintroducing it. The idea is to see whether symptoms get better and return when the milk is reintroduced. The same can be tried for a breastfeeding mother, although most children with milk allergy can be safely breastfed without the mother needing to restrict her diet.

Even if symptoms improve, cow's milk may then be gradually reintroduced over a period of one week. This is because symptoms may resolve spontaneously and not be linked to cow's milk at all. Without reintroduction, a child may be wrongly labelled as milk allergic.

Allergy specialist dietitian Carina Venter explains: 'We have no other 'test' to diagnose delayed type food allergies, other than elimination and reintroduction. The reintroduction phase may be concerning for families but the upside is we will ensure that we are only avoiding foods that are triggering symptoms.'

How much calcium does my child need?

'One cup of milk contains about 300mg of calcium, so that is usually what I aim for in an equivalent. It is also important to aim for a milk with added Vitamin D and Iodine. For Vitamin D, I aim for 3ug [micrograms] or more per cup and for Iodine, I just choose any that is fortified, as very few are.' – Carina Venter RD, allergy specialist dietitian

The British Nutrition Foundation guidelines recommend the following milligrams per day of calcium:

0–12 months	525mg per day
1–3 years	350mg per day
4–6 years	450mg per day
7–10 years	550mg per day

Males

11–18 years	1000mg per day

Females

11–18 years	800mg per day

Source: nutrition.org.uk

Egg allergy

Egg allergy is very much the commonest food allergy, especially if you include the significant number of children who are allergic only to runny egg but tolerate cooked forms. With this in mind, up to ten per cent of babies can be classified as having an egg allergy, even though some may never have a reaction due to not eating runny egg before the allergy resolves.

It often presents before the age of one and, while it can persist into teenage years and, far less commonly, adulthood, it has a very good chance of being outgrown. In fact, around 80 per cent of egg allergy resolves during early childhood – some as early as two years, and the average by age seven.

It is the food allergy most commonly associated with eczema and can cause a variety of symptoms: your child may have an immediate IgE-mediated allergy, with swelling, hives, an itchy mouth, as well as abdominal pain, vomiting, breathing difficulties and asthma. Occasionally symptoms may be delayed, and centre on gut problems including reflux, diarrhoea and constipation – but this is less common than with milk.

Egg allergy may be outgrown gradually, with well-baked egg often the first food tolerated (for example a carefully prescribed amount in a muffin) – moving on to less well-cooked egg, such as boiled egg, later.

As with milk, there is an 'egg ladder' of steps that would normally be followed. Your GP or dietitian may supervise, but if previous reactions have been severe, or there are multiple food allergies or additional ongoing issues with asthma or eczema, then this is best done under the supervision of a specialist allergy doctor, dietitian or nurse.

Generally, a hen's egg allergy means avoiding eggs from ducks, geese, quail and other birds too.

In foods, egg must be declared as an ingredient. As well as baked goods such as cakes, biscuits and breads, you may find it in patisserie, ice creams and desserts, sauces such as tartare sauce, mayonnaise or horseradish, in certain cheeses (e.g. Manchego or Grana Padano), as a fining agent in some wines (where it must be declared above certain amounts in wines from 2012 vintage onwards), in Royal Icing, fresh pastas, pancakes and sweets including jellies, marshmallows, Creme Egg, Chewits and nougat, and even in stocks and gravies. The key message is: check every label every time.

The so-called milk and egg ladders are 'reintroduction' plans, with steps of increasing tolerance. This is possible because, unlike other allergens, the proteins for milk and egg alter or 'break down' when cooked, and may be better tolerated when well baked.

If and when to start on the ladder should be an individual decision discussed in concert with your doctor or dietitian. Children who have severe or multiple allergies, or other troublesome allergic problems such as asthma or eczema, should not attempt this unless under specialist supervision. In IgE-mediated food allergy, they should not be attempted if skin prick or blood tests show no significant improvement since diagnosis. The ladder should also only be attempted when the child is well and thriving – and not within six months of a significant reaction.

BSACI allergy guidelines (see bsaci.org) note that children with mild egg allergy can often tolerate 'extensively heated egg products' such as cake. It may be useful to know whether they have achieved tolerance by school age as it means accidental exposure is less of a concern and avoidance becomes less onerous.

As egg allergy frequently resolves in stages, children who tolerate well-cooked egg may still react to raw or undercooked egg. Similarly, the milk ladder should be approached with great caution, and after seeking medical advice.

There is no good evidence that the ladder helps to increase tolerance, so this is not a reason to embark upon it. It is useful when an allergy is suspected to have been outgrown, and to allow the child to open up his or her diet and therefore avoid the need for greater vigilance.

Your doctor or nurse should be able to provide you with a written milk or egg ladder. You can find the BSACI-recommended milk ladder at <https://www.bsaci.org/guidelines/bsaci-guidelines/cows-milk-allergy/> and egg ladder at <https://www.bsaci.org/guidelines/bsaci-guidelines/egg-allergy-2021/>.

Tree nut allergy

Tree nuts are distinct from peanuts, which are actually a legume. They are in a different botanical category and include almonds, hazelnuts, walnuts, cashew nuts, pecans, Brazil nuts, pistachios and macadamia. If you are allergic to these nuts you should also avoid oil containing them. Despite having the word 'nut' in their name, coconut, chestnut, pine nut and nutmeg are *not* regarded as tree nuts.

There can be some cross reactivity between tree nuts – for example both cashew and pistachio share a similar botanical make-up and these allergies may go hand-in-hand; ditto pecans and walnuts.

If allergic to tree nuts generally, watch out for nuts and nut oils in toiletries and cosmetics. They may be listed by their Latin names, as follows:

Almond: *Prunus dulcis (sweet)* or *Prunus amara (bitter)* (also *Prunus amygdalus*)
Brazil: *Bertholletia excelsa*
Cashew: *Anacardium occidentale*
Hazelnut: *Corylus rostrata, Corylus americana* or *Corylus avellana*
Macadamia: *Macadamia ternifolia* or *Macadamia integrifolia*
Pecan: *Carya illinoinensis*
Pistachio: *Pistacia vera* or *Pistacia manshurica*
Walnut: *Juglans regia* or *Juglans nigra*

It used to be the case that anyone with an allergy to a particular tree nut or to peanut would be advised to avoid all nuts. This is no longer believed to be appropriate – latest research suggests that allergies are unlikely to extend to all tree nuts. The Pronuts study[4] found that children with one nut allergy can, on average,

---

4 'Defining challenge-proven coexistent nut and sesame seed allergy: a prospective multicentre European study', Brough et al, *Journal of Allergy & Clinical Immunology*, 2019. See: <https://www.jacionline.org/article/S0091-6749(19)31409-5/fulltext>

safely eat nine other nut types. Avoidance of all can significantly limit the diet and choices, and may even lead to decreased tolerance, meaning that a patient may end up developing an allergy to a tree nut they have unnecessarily excluded.

This is something to discuss with your doctor, who may recommend a hospital supervised oral food challenge to rule out allergy, allowing you to include more tree nuts in your diet (see Chapter 3).

Paediatric allergy consultant Dr Robert Boyle notes: 'Avoiding nuts you are allergic to does not usually place too many restrictions on the diet, but if you avoid all nuts it can become a significant burden for the young person with food allergy and their carers. My practice is to support young people with food allergy to confirm which nuts they are allergic to, and to safely try out the other nuts to give confidence about them.'

What about shea nut?

Shea nut is a commonly used ingredient in chocolates and cosmetics, and raises a lot of questions among those with nut allergy. Studies show that shea nut butter does not generally pose a risk to allergic consumers, including those with tree nut or peanut allergies. Meanwhile, when used in confectionery and cosmetics it is highly refined and therefore unlikely to include any protein residues – the allergenic component.

It may be sensible to avoid the use of shea nut products on broken or eczema-prone skin, given the potential risks of 'sensitization' shown with other foods, such as peanut. The theory is that if you introduce an allergen through the skin before you've eaten it, this can raise the chance of developing an allergy (see Chapter 5).

Peanut allergy

Possibly the most 'famous' allergy, peanuts are not a nut but a legume – closely linked to other legumes such as lentils, soya beans, chickpeas and peas (they all grow in pods).

Despite its reputation, peanut is not inherently more 'dangerous' than other nuts. Some people claim they cause more severe reactions than other foods, but in reality their prominence as a cause of severe reactions reflects the fact that peanut allergy is the commonest food allergy at the age when more severe reactions tend to occur: i.e. adolescence and early adulthood. Peanut may also be known by a range of other names – groundnut, monkey nut, beer nut, cacahuete, earthnut, goober nut or madelonas.

It is estimated that around two per cent, or one in 50, children is allergic to peanut in the UK. It tends to persist, although approximately one in five will outgrow their peanut allergy, usually during childhood.

Children with peanut allergy may have a slightly increased risk of allergy to sesame or lupin (a legume found in flour or seed form, and increasingly commonly in gluten-free foods), but this is something to discuss with your doctor. If your child has already been eating sesame and lupin with no issues then there is no need to cut them out.

In toiletries, some medicines and cosmetics, peanut may be listed by its Latin name, *Arachis hypogaea*.

Sesame allergy

It is possible to be allergic to any seeds, but sesame is the most common culprit. The incidence of sesame seed allergy appears to have risen fairly steeply over the past 20 years, possibly linked to its growing use, and is estimated to affect something like one in 100 people.

Unfortunately, it tends to persist in 80 per cent of cases. Everyone has their bugbear but I find sesame possibly the trickiest allergy to deal with – simply because those dastardly little buggers get everywhere. Freshly baked bread is out of bounds for us, because nestling alongside the lovely crusty baguettes and chewy bagels are sesame-scattered varieties.

Tahini and sesame oil are increasingly common. Find me a kids' party in north London that doesn't include hummus. And the 'electrostatic' nature of the seeds means they can cling to charged surfaces – so in food production, when sesame seeds are present, cross contamination is a real issue. Hence the warnings across so many baked supermarket goods.

There is some suggestion that whole sesame seeds may be better tolerated than when sesame is broken down into oils and pastes – possibly because they pass unbroken through the digestive system. Talk this through with your doctor. Studies are ongoing to determine whether it is possible to tolerate a few stray seeds, which could potentially open up new possibilities to those living with the allergy. Most children with sesame allergy can tolerate other seeds, but discuss this too with your doctor before trying them.

In toiletries look for the Latin *Sesamum indicum*, and in foods, while sesame has to be declared as an ingredient, remember to look out for tahini, halva and sesame oils.

Soya allergy

Soya allergy is less common in the UK compared to milk, egg, peanut, tree nut and fish allergies. There are limited stats but some estimates place soya allergy as affecting something like four in 1,000 children. Around one in ten children allergic to cow's milk will also react to soy although very often this allergy is outgrown.

As with milk and egg allergies, an allergy to soya may be immediate (IgE) or delayed (non-IgE). Soya is a legume (the soybean) but it doesn't usually follow that someone with a soya allergy will also be allergic to other legumes.

Soya can be tricky to avoid – it is contained in as many as 60 per cent of manufactured foods. Look out, for example, for foods such as edamame, miso, tofu, tempeh, soy flour, soy, Teriyaki and Worcestershire sauces and oil.

It may be found in a wide variety of products from cakes and chocolates to breads, processed foods and ready meals. Most people with soya allergy can tolerate soya lecithin, an emulsifier that contains very little soya protein, but discuss this with your doctor first. Both soya and soya lecithin have to be highlighted as an ingredient under allergy labelling laws.

Fun facts

In the UK, specific food allergies are often seen among communities that commonly eat those foods – for example fish allergy may be more common in Polish, West Indian or Bangladeshi and Bengali families; lentil allergy may be more prevalent in Indian families.

Meanwhile, kiwi allergy has been well studied and clearly began a few years after kiwi exports to the UK started in the 1980s. A similar pattern is likely with peanut, which was introduced to the UK by American soldiers around the time of the Second World War.

Legume allergy

There are suggestions – although currently limited data – that allergies to certain legumes are rising. It is more common to be allergic to chickpea, lentil and pea than to other beans such as string beans, kidney beans, black beans and so on. It's possible to be allergic to just one type of lentil, too – red lentil rather than green, for instance.

While there is a botanical link between peanuts and other legumes such as beans, lentils, chickpeas and peas, only about five per cent of children with peanut allergy will also react to any of these. There is no need to assume an allergy to any of these just because your child has a peanut allergy, but of course if they have shown symptoms when eating them, you should seek the advice of your doctor.

Another legume that can be potent as an allergen is lupin, most often found in processed foods, and in gluten-free breads and pastas.

It's incredibly frustrating for families of children with legume allergy that all of these foods are being used in increasing quantities in so-called 'free from' food manufacture. When our son was younger and allergic to wheat, egg, nuts, chickpeas, peas and lentils we found it virtually impossible to track down safe bread for him; at that time I think there was only one brand available in any of the supermarkets. Legumes are also used extensively, unsurprisingly, in vegan products.

There is also a tendency among non-allergic people to underplay the risks of something as seemingly benign sounding as a 'pea allergy'. Yet it is perfectly possible to have as severe a reaction to peas, or any other legume, as it is to milk, for example, or nuts.

Legumes other than lupin are not (yet) included in the list of 14 major allergens that food businesses have to emphasize by law, making avoidance that bit harder and reading labels vital (as it always is).

Other allergies

There are, of course, many more foods that children may be allergic to, some more commonly than others.

Fish allergy is frequently seen in children. Often, those with an allergy to one type of fish (cod, for example, or salmon) will also react to others as their proteins are similar. There is no evidence to suggest any associated increased risk of shellfish allergy.

Banana may present in infancy but is often outgrown by the age of two or three, and wheat allergy (as opposed to coeliac disease or wheat intolerance) may be seen in infants and pre-school children but is also often outgrown. There are, however, instances of persistent wheat allergy, usually along with rye, barley and oats.

Kiwi is another allergy believed to be on the increase. On occasion, allergies to banana or kiwi can be related to latex allergy, as can melon, avocado, chestnuts, pineapple, potato, papaya and passion fruit, but this is less common.

Sometimes, certain acidic fruits may aggravate the skin and cause a red rash around the mouth when eaten – such as strawberries or tomatoes and tomato-based sauces. However, if localized and not accompanied by any other symptoms, this is unlikely to be an allergy.

2

How to recognize and treat an allergic reaction

The most important tool in your allergy management toolkit (medicine aside, of course) is knowledge: being able to recognize the signs and symptoms of allergic reactions, and to know when and how to treat them. Similarly, helping your child to develop their own awareness and understanding of their allergy will pave their path to independence. Here goes for a rundown:

What is anaphylaxis?

'Anaphylaxis' (pronounced ana – fil – ax – is) comes from the Ancient Greek 'ana', meaning 'against' and 'phylaxis', meaning 'protection'. It is a severe and often sudden allergic reaction. Reactions usually begin within minutes and escalate but can rarely occur up to two to three hours later. It is potentially life-threatening and requires an immediate emergency response.

Common food triggers include milk, peanuts, tree nuts, egg, shellfish and sesame – although they are by no means isolated to the so-called 'Top 14' allergens (of which more later). Despite peanut being the most 'high profile' allergen, cow's milk is increasingly identified as a trigger for severe anaphylaxis, particularly in children.

Anaphylaxis can also be caused by drugs, wasp or bee stings and latex. In some rarer cases the cause is not known, which is termed 'idiopathic anaphylaxis'.

Despite the high profile of food-related anaphylaxis, only 30 per cent of UK hospital admissions due to anaphylaxis since

1998 are linked to food (others include drugs and insect stings) – and, while hospitalizations have increased, food-related fatalities have decreased over that time.

How do I know if my child is having an anaphylactic reaction?

As a general rule, a reaction that affects the airways, breathing or circulation is classed as a serious reaction, or anaphylaxis. The British Society for Allergy & Clinical Immunology (BSACI) presents an 'ABC' guide so you can better recognize the symptoms:

Any **one or more of the following** may be present:

A Airway

- persistent cough;
- hoarse voice;
- difficulty swallowing;
- swollen tongue.

B Breathing

- difficult or noisy breathing;
- wheeze or persistent cough.

C Consciousness/Circulation

- persistent dizziness;
- pale or floppy;
- suddenly sleepy;
- collapse/unconscious.

Other symptoms may occur alongside the 'ABCs'. These could include:

- widespread flushing or reddening of the skin
- hives – potentially spreading across the body

- swelling of the skin anywhere on the body (for example, lips or eyes)
- abdominal pain, nausea and vomiting.

These latter symptoms can happen on their own and be treated with antihistamine, but the patient should be closely monitored to ensure (a) symptoms do not escalate and (b) that the antihistamines have had an effect (typically within 30 minutes).

Resuscitation Council UK guidelines note that, 'although skin changes [such as hives or swelling] can be worrying or distressing ... skin changes without life-threatening Airway/Breathing/Circulation problems are not anaphylaxis. Reassuringly, most patients who present with skin changes caused by an allergic reaction do not go on to develop anaphylaxis'.[1]

One handy mantra often used is, 'antihistamine for hives, but adrenaline saves lives'.

As a side note, anaphylaxis and 'anaphylactic shock' are not the exact same thing. Anaphylactic shock is a consequence of an anaphylactic reaction and refers to a dramatic fall in blood pressure where the patient may become weak and floppy, and may also have what is often described as a sense of 'impending doom'. This can lead to collapse and loss of consciousness.

It's important to note that the risk of dying from an anaphylactic reaction from food remains very small. Studies show that, while hospitalizations in the UK due to anaphylaxis have increased threefold from 1998 to 2018,[2] there has actually been a decline in the case fatality rate for food anaphylaxis.

1 'Emergency treatment of anaphylactic reactions: Guidelines for healthcare providers', Resuscitation Council UK. See: <https://www.resus.org.uk/library/additional-guidance/guidance-anaphylaxis/emergency-treatment>

2 'Food anaphylaxis in the United Kingdom: analysis of national data, 1998-2018', Baseggio Conrado et al, *The BMJ*, 2021. See: <https://www.bmj.com/content/372/bmj.n733>

Based on data from 13 studies worldwide, researchers at Imperial College London also calculated that, for any person with a food allergy, the chance of dying from anaphylaxis in one year is 1.81 in a million. For children and young people aged 0–19, the risk is 3.25 in a million – compared to the risk of dying from accidental causes which, in Europe, is 324 in a million.[3]

This isn't to minimize the huge anxiety felt when living with allergy – sometimes these stats are used to imply we are exaggerating. The truth is that the stress lies in not being able to predict whether you or your child is at risk of the most serious reaction, and having to maintain the same levels of vigilance all the time in order to prevent a reaction from happening.

Anaphylaxis should always be treated as a medical emergency, not least because inappropriate or delayed treatment can contribute to the risk of fatality. The question is, how do we learn to manage and live with the risks, without severely disrupting quality of life?

How might a young child describe a reaction?

I can't remember where I found this list – it was probably pulled together from a few different places – but when my son started school I typed it out and it now forms part of the allergy care plan that I give to his new teacher every year.

Children don't always have the words or the understanding to know that what they are experiencing is a reaction. So these are some of the symptoms they may well describe:

- 'My tongue/mouth is hot/burning/tingling/itching'.
- 'There's a hair in my mouth'.
- 'My mouth feels funny'.
- 'My throat feels spicy'.
- 'There's something stuck in my throat'.
- 'It feels like there are bugs in there' (to describe itchy ears).

---

3 'Incidence of fatal food anaphylaxis in people with food allergy: a systematic review and meta-analysis', Umasunthar et al, *Clinical & Experimental Allergy*, 2013. See: <https://onlinelibrary.wiley.com/doi/epdf/10.1111/cea.12211>

I won't lie, we have had false alarms on one or two occasions. Like the time we had 'there's something stuck in my throat … oh, it's a bit of apricot.'

Or, 'it feels like there's a hair in my mouth! … actually there is.'

But it's always good to let others caring for your children know what to watch and listen out for.

Could my child react to airborne allergens?

The first and important thing to note is that it is uncommon to have reactions from simply being near to your allergens, and in those rare instances symptoms are usually mild. Being beside someone eating a peanut butter sandwich, for instance, would not pose an issue. It may be worrying to be able to smell your allergen – peanut butter in particular has a distinctive odour – but this doesn't mean any allergenic proteins are circulating.

To cause a reaction, the food protein has to be disturbed in a way that gets it aerosolized, or physically detectable in the air. This might happen where there are vapours from cooking – when milk is steaming, or where fish is frying, for instance, or where food in a powdery form is disturbed, such as flour. For an allergic person this can trigger symptoms including itchy eyes and a runny nose, or wheezing. It is highly unusual for air exposure to food proteins to result in a severe reaction. The chance of a reaction would also depend on how much protein gets into the air and how far away the allergic person is, as well as how large or airy the room is, and how sensitive the individual may be.

Some allergens more than others may be triggers for airborne reactions. Airborne reactions to peanuts, for example, appear to be much more rare.

However, this isn't to dismiss the likelihood – a recent study[4] showed that a small minority of children – two per cent – displayed

4 'Peanuts in the air – clinical and experimental studies', Bjorkman et al, *Clinical & Experimental Allergy*, 2021. See: <https://onlinelibrary.wiley.com/doi/10.1111/cea.13848>

mild symptoms (in this case, itchy, runny eyes and nose) when left in close proximity to a bowl of peanuts in a closed room. There were, however, no moderate or severe reactions reported.

Dr Hazel Gowland, an expert advocate, researcher and trainer in allergy risks, notes: 'I have heard credible anecdotes going back a long time – fish in the air from cooking, that sort of thing. One woman reported her throat closing after she went to a wedding where a cloth was dramatically swept off a buffet, wafting peanut into the air.'

Self-reported reactions can also be complicated by the fact that symptoms of anaphylaxis and panic attack may be very similar. The person may also have unwittingly come into contact with their allergen via other means – accidental ingestion, for example, after touching a contaminated surface. For some, significant anxiety may be caused by the perceived smell of an allergen they are avoiding.

It is sensible to be aware of your child and whether they react in certain situations. Some parents of children with milk allergy report mild reactions in coffee shops, for example, where milk vapours may be circulating. Or, as Dr Gowland notes, 'When you go to Granny's, your eyes are always swollen – so is that the cat? Is it something else? The best thing you can do is know your child well.'

I've heard people say their child is allergic to contact ... is that something I need to worry about?

For most people with allergies, coming into accidental skin contact with their allergen would cause only very mild reactions, such as redness or localized hives. Wiping the skin clean and giving a dose of antihistamine, if the rash is itchy, would usually clear the reaction promptly.

For parents of young children, especially babies and toddlers, contact is a bigger worry because of the risk their child may stick a hand in a smear of butter, for example, then transfer that hand to their mouth, or rub their eyes. This is why you'll find an allergy parent shuffling around like a latter-day Gollum before, behind and beside their kid mopping up any spills in sight and giving their grubby hands a frequent wipe.

Sometimes those allergens pop up where you least expect them – like the remnants of sticky broken egg in a hat box at a farm we once visited. I unwittingly stuck my hand in the box, then touched my son's arm, which broke out in a few hives where I had touched him. They were quickly resolved with a wipe clean and some antihistamine.

Many will have heard about the tragic story of 13-year-old milk-allergic schoolboy Karan Cheema, who died in 2017 after another child threw a piece of cheese at him. A review of this incredibly sad case by paediatric allergy specialists Dr Ru-Xin Foong, Dr Paul Turner and Professor Adam Fox[5] concluded that it was the first and only documented incident of its kind. A number of factors may have played a part, including uncontrolled asthma and eczema, delay in administering the EpiPen – with only one given despite no improvement in symptoms – and the fact that the AAI (Adrenaline Auto-Injector) was nearly a year out of date. The review concluded: 'We consider this case to be unique and unprecedented. It does not challenge standard advice that cutaneous [skin] exposure through non-denuded [non-damaged] skin is extremely unlikely to cause severe reactions.'

So, it is really important to be aware that casual contact is highly unlikely to cause any significant issues but – as a motto to keep throughout the allergy journey – it is always wise to keep on top of eczema outbreaks and be vigilant about avoiding contact with allergens when skin is broken.

---

5 'Fatal anaphylaxis due to transcutaneous allergen exposure: An exceptional case', Foong et al, *The Journal of Allergy & Clinical Immunology*, 2020. See: <https://www.sciencedirect.com/science/article/abs/pii/S221321981 9308499?via%3Dihub>

How do I treat an allergic reaction?

Treatment of a mild to moderate reaction

What is a mild to moderate reaction? The BSACI guidelines state swollen lips, face or eyes; itchy or tingly mouth; hives or itchy skin rash; tummy pain or vomiting; and sudden change in behaviour. In these instances, antihistamines are the first port of call.

The BSACI guidance is:

- Stay with the child, call for help if necessary.
- Locate adrenaline auto-injector(s).
- Give antihistamine.
- If vomited, can repeat dose.

Previously, so-called 'first generation' antihistamines were prescribed. These include brand names such as Benadryl and Piriton. In the past few years second generation antihistamines have become the preferred option – such as cetirizine. This is because 'first gen' antihistamines can cause more drowsiness, fatigue and impaired concentration. The second generation variants are widely regarded as less sedating and more efficacious. Children under two will often be prescribed Piriton, but talk to your doctor as they may be happy to offer a second generation alternative. This is particularly important if your child needs antihistamine regularly, as it can make them sleepy.

Keep up the fluids
If your child is having an allergic reaction, after administering their medication try to keep up their fluid intake by offering them plenty of water.

Treatment of anaphylaxis

Your child should be prescribed an AAI if they are judged to be at risk of anaphylaxis. You'll probably know an AAI by the most famous brand name – the EpiPen. But there are others, all of which operate in pretty much the same way (see below for detail).

Adrenaline (also known as epinephrine, hence 'EpiPen') is the first-line treatment for anaphylaxis, which should be seen as a 'first-aid measure combined with calling for emergency medical help'. It is not, despite how it may be portrayed in certain family movies we shall not name (*Peter Rabbit*), a magic 'one jab and you're fixed' solution. Essentially, it buys important time before a patient is able to receive proper medical attention.

The decision on whether to prescribe adrenaline should be based on several factors, including the causes of reactions, specialist assessment of severity and future risk, presence of asthma (which may increase risk) and the age of the patient. It is difficult – if not impossible – to accurately predict who is at risk of a severe reaction. According to the BSACI, it may include patients who:

- have suffered a severe reaction where the allergen cannot be easily avoided;
- are allergic to high-risk allergens, for example nuts or milk;
- cannot easily avoid the allergen;
- are at continued risk of anaphylaxis (e.g. those with food-dependent exercise-induced anaphylaxis);
- have idiopathic anaphylaxis;
- have significant co-factors (e.g. poorly controlled asthma).

The BSACI also states that 'prescribing an auto-injector cannot be a substitute for allergy referral'.

Importantly, a 2018 paper by paediatric allergists Dr Katherine Anagnostou and Dr Paul Turner[6] notes: 'Healthcare professionals must consider the patient/family preference: if

6 'Myths, facts and controversies in the diagnosis and management of anaphylaxis', Anagnostou et al, *Archives of Diseases in Childhood*, 2019. See: <https://adc.bmj.com/content/104/1/83>

prescription boosts patient confidence and allows them to lead a less restrictive life, then auto-injectors should be part of the management plan.'

It is also vital that anyone prescribed an AAI should receive:

- specialist advice on avoiding triggers;
- a written treatment plan;
- regular – ideally annual – retraining on the use of the AAI;
- referral to an allergy clinic.

The BSACI guidance adds that, in the event of a serious reaction (see 'ABC' symptom checker) you should:

- Lie child flat. If breathing is difficult, allow child to sit, ideally slightly reclining and with legs raised.
- Use adrenaline injector without delay.
- Dial 999 for ambulance and say 'ana-phy-laxis'.
- If after five minutes symptoms do not improve, give a second dose in the other leg.
- Do not stand, walk or sit up suddenly before emergency help arrives – changes in posture can worsen anaphylaxis.
- If the child carries an asthma inhaler and is wheezy, give the AAI first and then the asthma reliever (blue puffer).

US versus UK guidelines

At some point you will come across US-based advice on managing allergic reactions and it may send you into a spin. It's one of the issues that comes up most frequently in allergy groups and online forums. Whereas in the UK swelling of the face, hives, vomiting and tummy pain are classed as mild to moderate reactions, requiring antihistamine (and monitoring), in the US these are classed as anaphylaxis, requiring the EpiPen.

Many parents see US guidance – often as baldly put as 'anything more than hives, give epi' or to give epinephrine if you've eaten something you're allergic to, regardless of whether there are any symptoms – and it causes huge amounts of anxiety, confusion and uncertainty. 'How on earth will I know if my child is having an anaphylactic reaction if the advice differs so dramatically? Should I just give the EpiPen if I think he or she may have eaten something they're allergic to? What if these mild symptoms get worse?' Trying to make sense of it all is incredibly stressful.

So why does the guidance differ and should we worry that the UK is perhaps too relaxed?

As Dr Paul Turner notes in his paper 'The Emperor Has No Symptoms: The Risks of a Blanket Approach to Using Epinephrine Autoinjectors for All Allergic Reactions'[7], fatal food-induced anaphylaxis is 'very rare'. Also, the 'vast majority' of fatal reactions are due to 'substantial levels of exposure ... often with other significant co-factors' (such as asthma, or having also consumed alcohol). In many cases, less severe anaphylaxis may even resolve without treatment.

However, it's the unpredictability that is hard to manage – we don't know who is most at risk. Dr Turner argues that the 'trend to ... recommend immediate use of AAIs ... even in the absence of any allergic symptoms' or for 'non-severe symptoms' is highly problematic. He suggests that it may even be driven, in part, by commercial interests – that is, patient literature provided by the manufacturers of the AAI devices rather than evidence-based assessments.

The other worry is that using an EpiPen too early means you have nowhere to go if symptoms escalate. There are no studies to suggest that early use can prevent an escalation to anaphylaxis. It's a delicate balance, because it is, of course, important to use the EpiPen without delay when needed.

What's the answer? In short, it's being fully informed of all the symptoms, how to manage them, and what they mean.

Dr Turner says: 'Of course, we do encourage our patients to use their ... autoinjector if they have signs of airway/respiratory or cardiovascular involvement, or if they are uncertain what to do, because of difficulty in recognizing or identifying symptoms in themselves or in their child. We also advocate epinephrine use in the context of a rapidly progressing reaction. However, we do not advise patients to inject epinephrine for urticaria or angioedema [hives or swelling], because, if they occur in isolation or rather in the

---

7 'The Emperor Has No Symptoms: The Risks of a Blanket Approach to Using Epinephrine Autoinjectors for All Allergic Reactions', Turner et al, *The Journal of Allergy & Clinical Immunology In Practice.*, 2016. See: <https://pubmed.ncbi.nlm.nih.gov/27283056/>

absence of other symptoms or signs, they are nearly always minor, self-limiting symptoms.'

Blanket 'use your EpiPen regardless' advice may be well-meaning, he concludes, but 'food allergic individuals and their carers need to be provided with more constructive strategies and support than merely being told to "use your pen".'

Professor of paediatric allergy Professor George du Toit says: 'There's a simple rule I teach. Symptoms on the outside (hives and swelling) use antihistamine. On the inside (wheeze, low blood pressure) use Epi. Consider vomiting an "outside" symptom but intense, ongoing abdominal or uterine pain an "internal" symptom.'

FAQs

Is adrenaline harmful or dangerous?

Given by injection into the muscle of the outer-mid thigh, adrenaline is safe and starts to work within minutes. It opens up the airways, stops swelling and raises the blood pressure. To allow it to work most effectively, it should be administered as soon as anaphylaxis is suspected. Around ten to 20 per cent of patients report fleeting effects including anxiety, dizziness and headache – although these symptoms could also be due to the reaction.

If you accidentally inject yourself in the thumb or elsewhere (this can occasionally happen if the pen is held the wrong way round, for instance) then do seek medical help, as this can damage the tissue.

Is it true that each subsequent allergic reaction will be worse than the last?

No, it doesn't automatically follow that each reaction is worse than the one before, but the risk is unpredictable. Equally, a mild reaction does not guarantee the next one will also be mild. Unfortunately, there is no test that can measure your relative risk of a severe reaction, which is why avoidance of the food you are allergic to is vital, as is having your medication with you **at all times.**

A new research project[8] backed by the Food Standards Agency aims to gather data about people that have previously suffered – and recovered from – severe, life-threatening reactions to food. This will hopefully lead into studies to establish what may set them apart from those who have milder responses.

Can anything make an allergic reaction worse?

There are risk factors for a more severe reaction, which include:

- poorly controlled asthma;
- if you have, or very recently had, an infection;
- if you exercise vigorously just before or after contact with the allergen;
- if you are also suffering from airborne allergy symptoms, such as hay fever;
- if you are under significant stress;
- if you have been drinking alcohol;
- how much allergenic food has been consumed – the more you consume, the worse the reaction is likely to be.

How many AAIs should I carry?

The UK's Medicines and Healthcare Products Regulatory Agency (MHRA) states that those prescribed an AAI should carry **two with them at all times** for emergency on-the-spot use. This is important in case one device is broken or used incorrectly, or a second injection is needed before emergency help arrives.

As with many things related to allergy, medical opinion is not necessarily clear-cut. The BSACI recommends one device –

---

8 'Using NHS Data to monitor trends in the occurrence of severe, food induced allergic reactions', Food Standards Agency. See: <https://www.food.gov. uk/research/food-allergy-and-intolerance-research/using-nhs-data-to-monitor-trends-in-the-occurrence-of-severe-food-inducedallergic-reactions>

with an extra one for schoolchildren to be kept in school – on the basis that 'one dose is usually effective for most reactions'. The USA recommends two devices be prescribed.

The UK allergy charity, Anaphylaxis Campaign, backs the MHRA stance. Arguments in favour of always carrying two AAIs include delays in emergency help arriving – especially of concern when travelling or in a rural area – as well as the huge benefit to patients and their families in terms of confidence and reduction of anxiety to know there is a 'back-up' should the first dose go wrong. This cannot be underestimated, as the impact of food allergy on anxiety and quality of life can sometimes be debilitating.

Practise, practise, practise!

You should be shown how to use an AAI when you are first prescribed one, and be run through the process at subsequent appointments. If not, ask for a demo. It's important to know exactly how to use your pen correctly. An allergy specialist, the practice nurse at your local GP surgery or school nurse should be able to help.

Arm yourself with an AAI trainer pen to practise with at home – the manufacturers will provide these (see <epipen.co.uk>, <jext.co.uk>) – and encourage your child to practise, too. These trainer pens have no needle and can be reset for repeated use. When my son was a toddler, a fellow allergy parent kindly sent us a little homemade 'doctor's set' with lanyard, name badge and an EpiPen trainer pen to encourage him to play around with it. It helped to demystify the pen, and for him to become familiar with its workings.

Another top tip is to practise with an expired EpiPen on an orange. This one's best for adults, though – be very careful not to inject your hand. If you do, seek medical attention straight away. And don't eat the orange afterwards!

Which AAI should I have, and which size?

There are several types of AAI, the most widely known being the EpiPen. Others licensed for use in the UK are Emerade and Jext. Emerade was briefly subject to a recall in 2020 because of a defect in one component in a small number of pens. But the fault has been remedied and the device is available in the UK again.

They come in various sizes:

EpiPen: 0.15mg and 0.3mg
Jext: 0.15mg and 0.3mg
Emerade: 0.15mg, 0.3mg and 0.5mg

General advice for all AAIs is that a child should be moved on to a 0.3mg dose (an 'adult' AAI) when their body weight is more than 25kg. If a higher dose AAI is available, the advice is to transition to 0.5mg once body weight exceeds 60kg. Some clinics may recommend a move to a 0.5mg dose once a child's weight exceeds 45kg.

In the absence of 0.5mg auto-injectors, such as when Emerade was recalled, some doctors advise a double dose of a 0.3mg pen, i.e. giving two 0.3mg AAIs in quick succession for children over 45kg. But this is a question to discuss with your allergy specialist, as the MHRA has said a single 0.3mg EpiPen or Jext device is a suitable replacement.

The other potential benefit of Emerade is that the device has a longer needle length. Early studies suggest this may be useful for some patients, particularly adolescent and adult women who may have more soft tissue in the thigh area, making it harder to achieve an intramuscular injection. This is something you should also discuss with your doctor.

In the US and Canada a new audio device, the Auvi-Q (known as Allerject in Canada), is on the market. The Auvi-Q is a slim, credit card-sized device that has the ability to 'talk' you through the administration of the epinephrine. It too comes in 0.15mg and 0.3mg doses and its fans prefer the small size – easier to fit into a pocket or bag. One study[9] found that previously untrained people preferred use of the Auvi-Q over the EpiPen, with fewer errors made. It is not yet known whether

9 'Auvi-Q Versus EpiPen: Preferences of Adults, Caregivers, and Children', Camargo et al, *The Journal of Allergy & Clinical Immunology In Practice*, 2013. See: <https://www.jaci-inpractice.org/article/S2213-2198(13)00125-6/fulltext>

this device will become available in the UK, but it's definitely one to watch.

In time, it is hoped even more innovative alternatives will be produced – there has been research into epinephrine tablets given under the tongue, for example, although both funding and the dominance of the big AAI manufacturers remain a barrier.

The parachute theory

Paediatric allergy consultant Dr Mich Lajeunesse likes to talk his patients through the 'parachute theory' of carrying EpiPens.

'Most people think of the EpiPen, or AAI, as a barrier – they don't want to use the pens, they think about it as a hurdle or a place they don't want to go. I always say, think of it like falling out of a plane and opening your parachute: the sooner you open it the softer the landing is going to be.'

How soon is too soon, though? He adds: 'The way I teach my patients is the first symptoms usually happen while you are eating, those are initial symptoms, probably in the mouth and recognition that something isn't right. But if it starts extending to tight chest, an asthma attack, a tight throat or feeling really unwell then things are going in the wrong direction, so use the adrenaline.'

What should happen after I give adrenaline?

Always seek emergency medical help if an AAI is administered. Administer the first dose and call 999 immediately afterwards. If you have had anaphylaxis, you will need to be observed in hospital after you have recovered. This is because, in around 1 in 20 cases, a second 'wave' of symptoms can develop – known as a biphasic reaction.

Around half of biphasic reactions occur within six to 12 hours of the initial reaction. National Institute for Health and Care Excellence (NICE) guidelines advise that children under 16 should be admitted into hospital for observation, while those over 16 should be observed for six to 12 hours. The observation period will be decided by the treating doctor, and will depend on various factors including how quickly the patient responded to the first dose of adrenaline. The Resuscitation Council UK <resus.org.uk> has guidelines on in-hospital observation based on these various risk factors.

In the past, corticosteroids (an anti-inflammatory medicine) such as prednisolone have been used to prevent biphasic reactions. But their efficacy is not established and has never been tested in a randomized clinical trial.

Before discharge, you should be given information about anaphylaxis signs and symptoms, the risks of a biphasic reaction – and clear instructions to return to hospital if this occurs – and replacement AAIs if yours have been used. If you haven't already been referred to a specialist allergy clinic, you should be given information on how to go about this. If you have suffered anaphylaxis, but haven't been prescribed adrenaline, you should be discharged with AAIs, or a prescription for AAIs.

The following are quotes from people who have had to use an auto-injector:

'I gave my five-year-old daughter her EpiPen after she developed symptoms during a hospital challenge to milk. She had a persistent 'allergy' cough (it sounds different to a normal cough, like low throat clearing) and when they listened to her chest she had a wheeze. I was scared, as I hadn't used an AAI previously [but] it worked almost immediately. It's much easier to administer than you think. Using it taught me it really is a wonderful privilege to have the AAI, and to be given the chance to resolve allergic reactions.' – Clare Hussein

'I first used adrenaline on my son when he was 15 months old. He took a sip from another child's milk bottle and his airways started closing up. It wasn't like all his other reactions and I knew straight away that this was anaphylaxis. When the needle went in he let out a cry, but the adrenaline worked within seconds and by the time the ambulance arrived, he was breathing normally. I felt reassured that we knew how to use the injector and it had worked so well.' – Emma Amoscato

'When I first used my AAI it was really easy! I felt it working almost straight away and within minutes I was sitting up and my symptoms were getting better. To a child I'd say it might hurt a bit, like someone pinching you or poking you in the leg, but it's over really quickly. It doesn't hurt as much as getting a vaccine, hitting your funny bone or stubbing your toe! The medicine will work really fast and it will make you feel much better. It will all be over in seconds, so try not to worry' – Becca Turner

'We had practised with a trainer pen before, so my daughter knew exactly what to expect. Remove cap, push firmly into thigh, count together, 1 elephant, 2 elephants ... No tears, it was all very calm and uneventful really! Jess said it stung a bit and she felt a bit shaky after. By the time the ambulance arrived her breathing was back to normal' – Jo, mum to Jess, 7

'The first time I had to administer an EpiPen was mid-lockdown. Both Osian's dad and I were juggling working from home and homes-chooling. Distracted, I accidentally filled his favourite beaker with cow's milk. A few minutes later, Osian came downstairs, saying his milk "tasted funny". Alarm bells started sounding in my head.

Within five minutes Osian had become very spaced out. His eyes glazed over and he seemed to retreat into himself. He also developed hives on his trunk and arms, redness and swelling around his face, and was coughing when he breathed in. I asked him to sit on the floor because I needed to tell him something very important: I had made a mistake and given him the wrong milk, that he might start to feel poorly.

He listened with eyes wide as I told him I was very sorry for my mistake, that I would stay with him and watch him to make sure he was OK. I went into autopilot and administering the AAI didn't feel like the daunting prospect it always had. He did cry out when the needle went into his leg, but he stayed completely still, as we had always explained to him how important this was to avoid injury to his leg.

I rang for an ambulance as soon as the pen had been administered and, while I was talking to the call handler, Osian began to vomit.

He then sat quietly and we saw gradual improvement. By the time the crew came, he was able to chat with them.

I've now administered the AAI, I did it correctly and it did its job. Osian has experienced the reaction, knows how it and the AAI felt, and it's no longer a mythical thing that we tell him might happen at some point. I'd say to parents: trust your instinct – you know when your child is in trouble, so act when you need to. Make a note in your diary to regularly refresh your memory on your child's action plan and how to administer the AAI. This will definitely kick in if you need it. It will help you to feel calm and in control, which will in turn help your child not to panic.' – Sarah, mum to Osian, 7

What happens if I lose my allergy medication?

One sunny Sunday I was bundling the kids into the car for lunch at my parents', briefly plonking my bag beside the open door while I strapped one of them into their seat. In a flash, some rascal* (*substitute as appropriate) swiped it, with purse, keys ... and my son's EpiPen kit inside. I honestly wouldn't have had a clue how to go about getting a replacement if my sister, a doctor, hadn't told me to ring 111. They arranged for a prescription to be sent to a local pharmacy and I was able to pick up an emergency replacement within a couple of hours.

So how do you get new medication in a hurry?

If it happens within GP or clinic opening hours, contact your prescriber to arrange an emergency prescription.

If this isn't possible:

- See a local GP and ask for a prescription. Staff at an NHS walk-in centre may be able to arrange for you to see a GP.
- Ask a local pharmacist if they can provide an emergency supply of your medicine.
- Outside normal GP hours, call 111 to arrange an emergency prescription or visit <https://111.nhs.uk/>.

You can get medicine from a pharmacist provided you have been prescribed the medicine before. The pharmacist will probably need to see you face-to-face and must agree that you need the medicine immediately (which, in the case of an EpiPen, you do). They will also need evidence, if at all possible, that you have been prescribed that medicine before, and will need to be satisfied with the dose that they should provide you with.

In the case of an asthma inhaler, they will only be able to provide you with the smallest pack size.

Always keep an eye on AAI expiry dates. Handily, both EpiPen and Jext offer an expiry alert service. Head to their websites and fill out the quick online forms. You will then receive a text when they are due to expire.

3

Diagnosis: how to get it and what to expect

Sadly, very often the path to diagnosis can be fraught with difficulty, adding a huge burden of stress and anxiety on families battling to make sense of their child's symptoms and reactions.

We spent months firefighting our son's eczema, which he first developed at six weeks, seeking advice from midwives, health visitors, the GP and, finally, dermatology specialists. Firstly we were reassured that it was cradle cap, then, as it travelled down his forehead and on to his face and neck, we were told it was still seborrheic dermatitis (a condition that typically goes away at six to 12 months). By the time he was three or four months old his whole body was covered in a red, bumpy rash that sat stubborn beneath the oil slick of lotions we slathered him in. From the time he had his first, mystery reaction through to diagnosis, we had to fight to get answers. Current data is scarce but there is estimated to be only one consultant allergist per two million of the population in the UK,[1] and services for children are more scant than for adults, meaning waiting times can be lengthy and appointments hard to come by.

Many GPs are well informed but there is still a big gap in understanding, and often families are turned away or their symptoms dismissed or missed.

Paediatric allergy consultant Dr Mich Lajeunesse agrees that there is an 'unmet need' – both in terms of the numbers of

---

1 'Allergy: the unmet need – A blueprint for better patient care', Corrigan et al, *Royal College of Physicians*, 2003. See: <https://www.bsaci.org/wp-content/uploads/2020/02/allergy_the_unmet_need.pdf>

allergy specialists in the UK but also in knowledge and expertise among GPs and within primary care. He says: 'Allergy is something of a Cinderella speciality. Most people have had very little teaching about allergy in med school – although that's now changed – and you don't know what you don't know.'

But he adds: 'It is being addressed. What we need to do is make sure we have GPs and paediatricians who have enough knowledge to be able to manage the amount of food allergy that comes their way … to manage things like eczema and milk allergy. [They] often won't see the need for specialist training, and we are showing them how beneficial it is. People are engaging with this. We're changing attitudes.'

In the past five years, the Royal College of Paediatrics and Child Health (RCPCH) has established a training programme for doctors with an interest in allergy. There are also hopes for a series of intermediate clinics, midway between primary care and hospitals – although funding can be a barrier. On the flipside, just because something looks like allergy, it doesn't mean it *is* allergy. It's so important to get a proper diagnosis, not least because this is the path to proper management and also because, as paediatric allergy consultants Dr Robert Boyle and Dr Paul Turner of Imperial College London note in a 2021 BMJ article,[2] 'Food allergy does not just mean dietary restrictions and increased food costs, but can also impact on social activities and cause anxiety due to fear of potential reactions'.

Misdiagnosis can cause significant unnecessary stress. A 2008 study found that 34 per cent of three-year-olds were reported by their families to have had an adverse reaction to a food – whereas the actual rate was six per cent.[3] A baby with eczema,

2 'A food allergy epidemic… or just another case of overdiagnosis?', R. Boyle & P. Turner, *BMJ*, 2021. See: <https://blogs.bmj.com/bmj/2021/02/17/a-food-allergy-epidemic-or-just-another-case-of-overdiagnosis/>

3 'Prevalence and cumulative incidence of food hypersensitivity in the first 3 years of life', Venter et al, *Allergy*, 2008. See: <https://pubmed.ncbi.nlm.nih.gov/18053008/>

or cradle cap, does not necessarily equate to a child with food allergies, but persistent eczema with unexplained flare-ups can be an early warning signal. Don't be tempted to experiment by cutting out a major food, such as milk, because this could lead to your child not getting the nutrients they need. Please do talk to your health visitor or GP, who may refer you to an allergy specialist or registered dietitian. If you aren't getting anywhere, refer to the NICE guidelines on paediatric food allergy diagnosis, set out in the section below.

The following are quotes from people about the wait to get a diagnosis:

'My son started vomiting at about a month old. Everyone told us it was just reflux. He didn't sleep well, either, but that's common in newborns. At around five months, when we began weaning, he developed severe eczema and was still vomiting a lot after milk feeds. The GP kept saying it was reflux and wouldn't refer us. I decided to use my work medical insurance to self-refer to a paediatrician. She too told me it was reflux and that my anxiety was making his eczema worse.

It was heartbreaking to see my son in his state. I asked the paediatrician to get some allergy blood tests done, which when they came back showed possible allergies to a range of things, including nuts, milk, sesame and eggs. At that point, she finally referred me to an allergist and a dermatologist.

Within two weeks of receiving a diagnosis and a management plan, his skin finally cleared. We were put on a prevention regime of a wash, ointments and steroid creams where necessary. We continue with his allergist who has put him on studies that involve food challenges and also immunotherapy. Zeke grew out of his milk allergy quickly and loves it now. He is still allergic to egg, for which we carry EpiPens.' – Anjuli Davies, mum to Zeke, 3

'I struggled tremendously breastfeeding Avi. He vomited a lot and his skin in the first few weeks seemed to be getting worse. Health *visitors put it down to baby acne. At three months his skin got so bad it was weeping and he started getting eczema around his neck and tummy. He was put on antibiotics as he had a skin infection. I spoke to the GP about a possible cow's milk allergy but they were dismissive.*

At six months, when I first weaned Avi, I gave him a rusk and seconds after him consuming this his voice went croaky, he was trying to cry but couldn't, this enormous bump formed on his head and little hives popped up everywhere. We took him to A&E and they immediately administered adrenaline. That was the day that changed everything for us.

We were told, after looking at his IgE levels, that we must avoid wheat, dairy, egg and nuts. We transferred to an allergy clinic and felt like we were getting somewhere, especially as the appointments were consistent. If I could go back in time I would push for an allergy test and wouldn't be fobbed off with lotions and potions. Had we known he had allergies we could have avoided an anaphylactic reaction. Go with your gut feeling and don't take no for an answer.' – Jasmine, mum to Avi, 6

Edel and Noah's story:

'Our son is nine and allergic to egg, peanuts, tree nuts and kiwi. When he was born he had some patches on his face which got progressively worse so, by the time he was eight weeks, he basically looked like he was covered in burns. The only part of his body not affected was his nappy area. He was sleeping in 20 minute bursts because his skin was so sore, yet my GP kept telling me to moisturize him, it was normal, and I was just an over-worried new mum.

I was contacting my doctor's surgery every few days about his skin, how he was crying and I knew something was wrong. I kept being dismissed. I took him for his 12-week vaccines and, just beforehand, our son scratched the eczema on his face. He was bleeding badly and really inconsolable. The doctor took one look at him and shouted at me. He told me my baby was suffering, that I should have brought him in sooner. I told him to check my notes, that he'd been seen almost weekly by a doctor and each time I'd been patronised and told I was being a worrier. And I just wept.

I could see he was furious with his colleagues. He put his arm around me and promised he would help. That man is the reason our son was diagnosed early and he personally ensured that for the next few months I saw him as our GP. He was wonderful. That day he phoned the dermatology department and, despite a waiting list of around 12 months, he stayed on the phone until they agreed to see him in five days' time.

He told me he thought it was a milk allergy, that he'd give me prescription milk and that dermatology would treat the eczema and refer our son to the allergy clinic. He was the first healthcare person in three months to listen and see that something was wrong.

The biggest issue is dismissing parent concerns as 'new mum paranoia'. I knew something wasn't right and no one would listen. We were lucky we met that GP at 12 weeks. Others might not be. Second opinions, private consultations etc. shouldn't be needed.'

What can I expect?

The National Institute for Health and Care Excellence (NICE) guidelines are evidence-based recommendations developed by independent committees. Their role as an organization is to improve standards and outcomes for people using the NHS, public health and social care.

NICE[4] guidance states that food allergy should be considered in children and young people who have one or more of the signs and symptoms of possible food allergy. These include:

- Diarrhoea or vomiting
- Wheezing and shortness of breath

---

4 'Food allergy in under 19s: assessment and diagnosis', NICE. See: <https://www.nice.org.uk/guidance/cg116/ifp/chapter/Person-centred-care>

- Itchy throat and tongue
- Itchy skin or rash
- Swollen lips and throat
- Runny or blocked nose
- Sore, red and itchy eyes
- 'Colicky' abdominal pain
- Eczema that doesn't respond adequately to treatment.

Signs of Non-IgE mediated allergy also include:

- Eczema
- Loose or frequent stools
- Blood and/or mucus in stools
- Food refusal or aversion
- Constipation
- Pallor and tiredness
- Faltering growth plus gastrointestinal symptoms.

If food allergy is suspected by the family or by a healthcare professional, a GP should take a full, allergy-focused history of the patient. This includes:

- any personal history of atopic disease (asthma, eczema or hay fever, for example);
- any family history of atopic disease or food allergy;
- details of the food suspected and why;
- questions about when symptoms first started, speed of onset; following food contact, how long symptoms persist, how severe they are, where they take place.

If your healthcare professional suspects that your child might have an allergy to one or more foods, they should first give you and your child some information about food allergies, including the type of allergy they think it could be (see definitions in Chapter 1), whether there is risk of a severe reaction and how the allergy can be properly diagnosed. They should also give you information about where to find support, including how to contact support groups.

If your child has a suspected cow's milk allergy (CMPA) you should be offered advice about what type of hypoallergenic formula to use for a bottle-fed baby, or what type of milk substitute to use for an older child. Breastfeeding mothers should be given advice about what – if any – foods to personally avoid. You should also be offered help from a dietitian if you need it.

What next? How a food allergy is diagnosed

Skin prick tests and blood tests

If your doctor suspects an IgE-mediated food allergy, they should offer either a blood test or a skin prick test (SPT).

In a skin prick test, a drop of liquid containing the suspected food protein is placed on the forearm, and a tiny prick is made in the skin through the drop to see if a reaction occurs. This would take the form of a hive, or a 'wheal and flare' – a raised bump surrounded by some redness – and would typically show after 15 to 20 minutes. The allergy nurse or doctor will measure the size of that wheal and flare, which will help them to assess whether it is a 'positive' or 'negative' result. As a very general rule, anything over 3mm or 4mm could be considered a positive response. This means the patient is sensitized to that food, although doesn't automatically signal an allergy. The results may also differ depending on the food – for example a 2000 study[5] posited that a predictive positive for milk allergy would likely be above 8mm, for egg above 7mm and for peanut above 8mm. The bigger the size, the more likely you are to be allergic – but size does not predict the severity of a reaction.

---

5 'Specificity of allergen skin testing in predicting positive open food challenges to milk, egg and peanut in children', Sporik et al, *Clinical & Experimental Allergy*, 2000. See: <https://pubmed.ncbi.nlm.nih.gov/11069561/>

There will also be a 'positive control' and a 'negative control'. The positive control is usually a drop of histamine solution, and this will break out into a hive and become itchy. The negative control is usually a saline solution, which should trigger no response. The negative control is important because it excludes the presence of dermographism – where the skin naturally 'flares' when scratched, which, if present, makes the tests difficult to interpret. Generally, a commercially-produced solution for a wide range of allergens is used, but for some foods more accurate results are achieved if the fresh product is used. For example, your clinic may use tahini when testing for sesame, or crushed lentils or chickpeas.

A blood test, meanwhile, looks for the presence of antibodies to the allergen in the blood. You may hear these tests described as RAST (radioallergosorbent) tests. They are more expensive than skin prick tests and the results have to be analysed by a lab, so take longer. On the plus side, it is a good way to test for multiple allergies at once. They may also be recommended if the skin is very broken or sensitive. Again, the higher the levels reported back the greater the likelihood of allergy – but these **do not predict the severity of any reaction.**

These tests are both similarly reliable and a decision on which is done will depend on local services available. It's vital to note that the results are not definitive – **no test is 100 per cent accurate and no skin prick or blood test alone is enough to diagnose allergy.** There are a lot of false positives: for example, 40 to 80 per cent of positive IgE results for peanut occur where no allergy exists.[6] These people would get a positive result to a skin prick test but would not react when peanuts are consumed. A positive result from one of these, along with a documented history of symptoms, would often be enough to confirm allergy.

6 'Sense About Science: Making Sense of Allergies', 2015. See: <https://www.immunology.org/sites/default/files/making-sense-of-allergies.pdf>

Antihistamines, if not avoided for two days (for short-acting antihistamines such as chlorphenamine) or five days (for long-acting antihistamines such as cetirizine or loratadine) before a skin prick test, can also lead to inaccurate results, as the antihistamine may suppress any reaction. Your allergy nurse or doctor will ask if any have been taken before conducting the tests. 'Blanket' allergy testing for multiple allergens is not generally recommended as it can give false positive results and lead to unnecessary dietary restrictions.

Tests are not enough

A skin prick test or blood test must be carried out alongside a thorough history of the patient, including information on previous reactions, symptoms and more. **A blood or skin prick test alone is not enough to either diagnose or rule out allergy.** It is one in an armoury of tools the allergy specialist will use to figure out whether your child has a food allergy. Allergists are rather like detectives – they examine the evidence and pick up on often complex clues to reach a diagnosis.

You should not be left with the results of a skin prick or blood test with no accompanying explanation of what those results mean, or what action you should take to manage a suspected food allergy. If this happens, you should ask to see your doctor again to discuss the results in full.

Diagnosing non-IgE-mediated food allergy

There are no tests to measure non-IgE-mediated food allergy, i.e. those symptoms and reactions that may occur hours or even days after eating certain food. You will very likely be advised to keep a food diary and to try an elimination diet under the supervision of a nurse, doctor or dietitian. This means avoiding the suspected food for a period of up to six weeks, before reintroducing it. This could involve one or several foods. If the symptoms return when that food is eaten again, it may confirm the allergy.

If you are advised to try an elimination diet, you should be offered help and advice, including how to understand food labels to ensure your child doesn't eat the food by mistake, what foods to substitute to ensure they are getting a healthy balanced diet, and how to reintroduce the food safely.

Alternative tests for food allergy

You may have heard or been told about high street or DIY tests to diagnose your child's food allergy. These include 'food intolerance tests' or 'IgG antibody tests', applied kinesiology, hair analysis and Vega tests. There is **no evidence** that they can diagnose food allergy.

Unfortunately, many of the people offering these tests can be convincing. They can have big name celebrity backers, pop up first on a Google search, gain press coverage and airtime, and can also exploit the anxiety many parents feel when faced with a baffling array of symptoms – and sometimes difficulty getting a diagnosis. It's understandable that, when feeling desperate, worried and unable to find help, families might turn to other sources. However, I'm going to be blunt here: these tests are a waste of your time and money. At worst, they could lead to you cutting out vital foods from your child's diet unnecessarily – leading to malnutrition.

If you are really struggling and at your wit's end trying to get diagnosed, please contact one of the allergy charities for advice: the Anaphylaxis Campaign and Allergy UK contact details are at the back of this book.

In the Sense About Science factsheet '*Making Sense of Allergies*', consultant paediatrician Dr Paul Seddon says: 'These dubious tests, like IgG tests and the hair test, lead consumers and patients to believe they are getting an accurate diagnosis of their allergies. The NHS Choices website says these tests are 'less reliable' – but in fact they are worthless.' He adds that these false diagnoses can cause both physical and psychological harm, such as children being wrongly led to believe they are in danger if they eat certain foods, as well as being placed on 'inappropriately restricted diets, often for many years, and without either dietician advice or review of diagnosis'. He says: ' This can lead ... to lack of calcium intake, iron deficiency, or poor growth and weight gain.' Dr Seddon adds: 'I don't know why companies are permitted to continue to advertise "allergy tests" which have no scientific basis.'

More recently, companies have sprung up offering IgE tests (skin prick and blood tests) for allergy – the type of blood test you may be offered in hospital. However, even though the technology itself may be sound, they still throw up huge risks. Experts describe them as a 'recipe for misdiagnosis'. These companies often hide behind the disclaimer that results should be interpreted by a doctor – but given people using them will have bypassed a doctor already, this is highly unlikely to happen.

As the American Academy of Allergy, Asthma & Immunology points out in its list, 'Ten Things Patients and Physicians Should Question' (this one's at number one): 'Don't perform ... an indiscriminate battery of IgE tests in the evaluation of allergy. Appropriate diagnosis and treatment of allergies requires ... the patient's clinical history.'

Dr Dave Stukus, a US paediatric allergy specialist known for his myth-busting on social media, writes: 'I see the allure. On the surface, it seems great. A simple blood test to screen for more than 100 food allergies ... just to see if anything pops up. Unfortunately, that's not how it works. The truth is, these panels cause real harm. They lead to misdiagnosis. They force unnecessary avoidance. They make people have real anxiety about food allergies that don't even exist. In some cases, they actually create food allergy in someone who is sensitized but tolerant, and then avoids for a period of time. I meet people every day whose lives are turned upside down by these tests. Avoid the marketing. Avoid the Instagram influencers promoting these tests. Avoid unnecessary angst and avoidance.'

When you should see a specialist

If an elimination diet has not worked, your child has been judged to have had a severe reaction, or if they have asthma or persistent atopic eczema as well as allergies, you should be referred to an allergy specialist. You may also be referred if the results of your child's allergy tests are negative but your healthcare professional still suspects food allergy – or if they are allergic to more than one food.

Find an allergist

If you're not sure how to find a genuine allergy specialist, the BSACI Find a Clinic tool on their website is hugely helpful <https://www.bsaci.org/workforce/find-a-clinic/>. You will still need to be referred by a GP but it offers a comprehensive list of all UK clinics. If you find yourself needing to see an allergist privately, choose one who also currently works in the NHS.

Handy questions to ask your doctor

- What type of food allergy do you think my child has?
- What tests are you proposing and why?
- How long will it take to get the results, and will I have a follow-up appointment to discuss those results?
- Should I avoid the foods completely?
- Why have you come to this conclusion?

What to do if my child is nervous about skin prick tests?

Some kids blithely sit through a battery of skin prick tests (SPTs) with barely a flinch. Until he was about three or four, my son seemed largely unbothered, with maybe an extra blink or two. As he started to get more aware, he got more nervous and reluctant. I'd have to sit him tightly on my lap and hold his arm in place. The nurses kindly put the TV on to distract him.

I'd always buy him a comic from the hospital shop on the way out, as a little bit of bribery and reward.

Sometimes children can be so fearful or nervous that they refuse to have the tests, or panic at the last moment. Clare Hussein, whose daughter developed a fear of SPTs at the age of six, came up with a system to help coach her through it. 'What worked for us was writing down each small step and giving her a sticker when she completed each one – sitting in the chair, then putting her arm on the pillow, then allowing the nurse to write on her arm and so on. She'd then get a certificate at the end. We also agreed that the drops of allergen and the physical skin prick wouldn't go ahead until she said a pre-decided word that she had chosen. It helped her with feeling in control. This was also broken down into each single drop or prick. Involving her helped loads, as well as chatting about what was wrong or why she was scared ... even if she didn't really know.'

Paediatric allergist Professor George du Toit adds: 'Children are frequently anxious prior to skin prick testing, so you need a calm, informative and playful professional approach, and this includes nurses, doctors and even welcoming clinic staff. Stick with a simple explanation; graphics and videos can also help. Sometimes we find doing it on the parent first or drawing shapes on the child's arm prior to skin prick testing – such as 'dot dot dot' caterpillars – frequently helps. Also, it might be a good idea to do the positive control last as this is usually the itchiest – and raw egg, as that's itchy too.'

Bringing along a favourite soft toy or doll can help, as a comforter. The nurses can also pretend to give the toy a skin prick test. Colouring books are another favourite – don't forget to ask for the skin prick test to be done on the opposite arm your child uses to colour! Similarly, listening to music or watching a favourite programme on a tablet (don't forget headphones) can be calming and soothing.

The Evelina London at Guy's and St Thomas' has some great allergy resources online, which you can find at:
<evelinalondon.nhs.uk/our-services/hospital/allergy-service/patient-leaflets.aspx>.

They recommend:

- Prepare for the day by calmly explaining to your child what will happen. Reassure them that this is a completely normal procedure.
- Plan a little reward for afterwards – whether that's buying a favourite comic or treat or visiting a playground. The Evelina recommends using 'now' and 'then' statements, such as: 'Now we will see the nurse, and then we will go for your treat.'
- Have lots of distractions for during and after the test – afterwards is when they may get itchy.
- Feeding may be comforting for breastfed babies, so consider saving a feed for the test if possible.

They also suggest describing a skin prick test as a 'bubble pop test'. Explain it as follows: 'First the nurse will write some numbers or letters on your arm, then they will put some tiny bubbles next to each number or letter, then the bubbles will be popped using something called a lancet, a bit like a toothpick'.

Clinical psychologist Dr Rebecca Knibb adds: 'I think preparing children and talking them through it all beforehand can really help with anxiety and nerves. Avoiding something usually makes anxiety worse. Parents will know best regarding what their children will understand and how they might explain what will happen. If parents are unsure themselves, I would urge them to talk to their doctor first, so they know what will happen. This can also reduce a parent's anxieties which will help the child, who may pick up on a parent's worries.'

It is very rare to have anything other than itchiness and redness following a skin prick test. These usually settle after a few hours, and can be eased with an ice pack or a dose of antihistamine. Very occasionally, a child may feel a little dizzy and need to lie down, but such a response would typically occur at the clinic where hospital staff will be on hand to help.

Oral food challenge

This is a 'don't try this at home' one. Well, it's a 'don't try this at home unless your allergy specialist explicitly tells you it's OK' one.

The basic premise of a food challenge is to try the suspect food allergen in incremental doses, under careful and constant monitoring, to see if there is any reaction. You can run a battery of blood and skin prick tests but the absolute gold standard, rock solid way to know for sure whether you have a food allergy is to, well, see if you react when you eat it. That's why, if skin prick tests, for example, result in a positive reaction to a food, if you are already eating that food without any symptoms you should carry on as normal. Quite clearly this is not something that you should undertake without medical advice or supervision. But the food challenge can be a hugely helpful tool.

If an allergy has been confirmed by a combination of a child's history and test results, a food challenge will not be performed. It may be suggested when results are borderline, or when it is suspected that an allergy has been outgrown. Paediatric allergy consultant Professor George du Toit explains: 'A supervised challenge is the gold standard test for the diagnosis of food allergy or tolerance. Oral challenges are most commonly performed when a patient's history isn't certain enough, either of allergy or tolerance.'

There is always the chance your child will not be able to tolerate the food, and may have a reaction, as between 20 and 50 per cent of patients do. But performed in a hospital setting, these challenges are supervised by highly-trained medical staff, who will monitor your child constantly and will stop the challenge if they think any symptoms may be developing.

We've been through dozens of food challenges now, since we set out on the allergy journey. We've been allowed to challenge foods at home when the doctor has been confident that our son has outgrown an allergy – wheat, back when he was two or three years old, and later walnuts and hazelnuts.

We've also had challenges in the hospital, which have gone both ways. Over the years we've been able to confirm that he has outgrown banana, lentil, pea, chickpea and tree nut allergies. We've been able to move him from a strictly no egg diet on to being able to eat specific quantities of well-baked egg. On the other hand, we had his sesame allergy confirmed when he reacted after the first dose during a challenge. He broke out in spreading hives and the challenge was stopped. We had our hopes dashed when he nearly made it to the finishing line with peanut – we actually got as far as the last dose and were on the cusp of being discharged when he started sneezing, then his eyes started watering and became swollen. So near and yet so far! And we didn't get to the end of the baked egg challenge on the first attempt: it took us two or three goes over a couple of years before he finally made it without tummy ache or hives.

It can feel hugely nerve-wracking to subject your child to a food challenge when you've worked so hard for so long to avoid that allergen. But I always say that it's worth it – whether we've been successful, or not. When successful it can be truly life-changing: it opens up a world of possibilities, new foods to be tried, a loosening of the blanket of anxiety that envelops you whenever you are around food. It's one less thing to worry about, one more thing to introduce. Even when unsuccessful, it's been hugely helpful too. We've seen how different foods spark different reactions – tummy ache for egg, swelling and sneezing for peanut, crazy all-over hives for sesame. We can recognize the gamut of reactions and our son can, too. We can see how reactions can be swiftly dealt with: so far we've only needed antihistamine during food challenges to stem a reaction. And we've been able to go away armed with more information about what he is allergic to and how we should deal with it.

A 2010 study[7] showed that parents of children with suspected peanut or hazelnut allergy had high levels of anxiety about a potential reaction. After the challenge, the anxiety was 'significantly lower', even in the group where a challenge had led to a positive allergy diagnosis.

All this said, be prepared for a long day followed by grumpiness if you're undergoing a food challenge. Typically, you will arrive to be assessed by an allergy nurse, quizzed over eczema and their general health, and they will check that you haven't taken any antihistamines in the past few days. Challenges aren't advised either if your child is unwell, as this can raise the risk of reactions, or, if they have a rash or runny nose, it may make deciphering a reaction harder. Their asthma will also need to be under control.

The food is then brought to you in carefully measured doses, starting with the tiniest amount. You wait 20 minutes and are checked over by the nurses, before the next, slightly bigger, dose is given. Sometimes the process can take hours, followed by a one or two-hour wait following the final dose, to be sure there is no delayed reaction. Even after passing a food challenge, you will be advised to go home and monitor for any delayed symptoms, and to avoid the food until 48 hours have passed. After that, you will be advised to give the food to your child at least three times a week to keep their tolerance going.

If your allergist advises you are OK to go ahead and challenge a food at home, but this is making you too anxious, consider

---

7 'Parental anxiety before and after food challenges in children with suspected peanut and hazelnut allergy', Zijlstra et al, *Paediatric Allergy & Immunology*, 2010. See: <https://onlinelibrary.wiley.com/doi/abs/10.1111/j.1399-3038.2009.00929.x>

asking if they will book an appointment to have it done in hospital instead. I know parents who have gone ahead and challenged in hospital car parks or outside GP surgeries, but if you are genuinely nervous, rather than skipping it please talk to your allergist about how you feel and see if something else can be arranged.

Mixed nut challenges

Sometimes, instead of challenging to one nut at a time, clinics may recommend mixed nut challenges where several types of nut are baked into a cookie, for example. This won't be suitable for all children, and it's a decision for your allergy clinic to make.

It can be useful for children for whom skin prick tests suggest they are not sensitized, but who are scared to introduce nuts at home. It can also be helpful for children with a low grade sensitization to all nuts – low skin prick tests for example. If one nut is higher on testing than the rest, this can be taken out of the mixed nut challenge.

Stories from the food challenge frontier:

'Food challenges feel unnatural because you're feeding them food they may be allergic to, but it's always so well controlled in hospital. Given it's the only true way to tell if a person is allergic I would recommend them if they are possible, because it gives you the best picture of what is happening and you can deal with the allergies in a more informed way.' – Clare Hussein

'My son Ola was eight when we had a controlled egg challenge. I had to prepare a muffin to the hospital's recipe and the idea was that he would consume small, carefully measured amounts a bit at a time. He had three-quarters of it and started to feel sick. He vomited quite a lot and we haven't tried him with egg since. For us, it was good to know and, for him, it was an experience that has now stopped him from even trying to sneak a bite at any food containing egg' – Sola Tayo

'My daughter, Martha, is now three. She was diagnosed with CMPA and egg allergy at six months. At age two, we were invited to a baked milk challenge as her numbers on skin prick tests were reducing – and she passed it. It was reassuring being in hospital, as I felt well supported by the nursing staff. The challenge was helpful for me emotionally as a parent – I began to believe that outgrowing her allergies was a real prospect. She's recently had her skin pricks again, and it now shows negative to milk. We're now on the milk ladder and about to move on to cheese – this is such an exciting step! I would advise families going through a food challenge that the hospital is a very safe setting and the nurses are wonderful and are used to this process. It's definitely worth it.' – Hannah

How do I explain a challenge to my child?

When my son had his first baked egg challenge, at the age of three, we really struggled with how to frame it. I went through the scenarios:

Scenario 1: Tell him we are trying a muffin with egg in it
The possible outcomes are:

1 He is nervous and refuses, the mantra 'no eggs' having been drilled into him since before he could walk.
2 He isn't tolerant of baked egg and has a reaction. OK, he'll then know exactly why eggs are bad, but will he trust us with any future food trials again?
3 He completes the challenge. Now he can have very specific amounts of baked egg but 'eggy' egg (e.g. scrambled, fried, etc.) remain no-nos. Can a three-year-old really assess the complexity of this scenario? Should a three-year-old have to assess the complexity of such a scenario? Might the still-present danger of eggs be lost on him after this?

Scenario 2: Don't tell him this is an egg challenge, just say we are trying a 'new cakey thing'
The possible outcomes are:

1 He reacts, and is then nervous about any future challenges we try.
2 He doesn't react, is none the wiser (for now) but we can introduce baked egg secretly and hope that this early tolerance develops into an outgrown allergy by the time he hits teendom.

In the end, we went for Scenario 2, figuring that at three he was too young to have to grapple with the intricacies of his allergies. 'The simpler we can make it for him, the better, and the safer,' I said to myself.

That'll teach me. First dose down and the allergy nurse came rocking up with a cheerful smile, the second dose ready in a pot and a booming, 'Here's your egg!'

What I learned from that little saga is it's probably, on the whole, best to be upfront and clear from the get-go. He wasn't able to tolerate the egg on that occasion, and we had to stop the challenge when he developed a tummy ache. But the positive outcome was that he now understood much better why he couldn't eat egg and what being allergic might mean. His early reactions had happened when he was a tiny baby, of which he obviously had no recollection.

Clinical psychologist Dr Kate Roberts says giving your child all the information they need is important: 'In most situations children can be a bit more aware than maybe we realize. The first step is understanding what your child is worrying about, making sure they have all the info they need at that point in an age appropriate way, perhaps gradually allowing them to take more responsibility. Let them ask questions or share worries.'

'We don't want our kids to grow up too fast but there's a point, even when they are little, that we need to realize their capacity to process and understand serious issues, like allergies. My son deals better with information about his allergies than my parents do. Keep it factual, be honest, caveat the scary with positives – for example, OK, you may have a reaction but you have your EpiPen and we all know what to do to keep you safe. Kids want to feel safe more than anything. It's hard to remove the emotion, especially when it's so overwhelming for parents, but it's what you need to do to keep them safe and build emotional resilience' – Edel

What if my child is too nervous or fussy to eat the challenge food?

It's little surprise that, after being told to 'avoid, avoid, avoid', some children baulk at the idea of eating food they believe they are allergic to. Children may be nervous, worried, confused or simply dislike the look, smell or taste of the food in question.

If you are facing this issue, speak to the clinic team before your visit to talk through the sort of foods your child does like – they may be able to adapt the challenge recipe to accommodate this. Similarly, it may be possible to mix the challenge dose with food your child enjoys.

Other tips include bringing a book, a tablet or activity that can help take your child's mind off the task. Some clinics have play therapists on site to alleviate anxiety and offer distraction techniques. You might also take along some of your child's favourite food to eat after they have had the dose – check with your clinic that this is allowed.

One parent recalls: 'A lovely nurse wrote my daughter's name in chocolate syrup on almond butter on a cracker for her (successful) almond challenge. Kind, patient nurses have always made a big difference.'

For more complex issues relating to feeding, ask for guidance from your local Speech and Language Therapy team, or a specialist feeding therapist. Speak to your allergy clinic about this, or ask your GP for a referral. It's also important that you are given written information about what to expect before, during and after the challenge so you can prepare your child.

Mind your language

One barrier to managing the minefield of food challenges – and skin prick tests for that matter – can be the language used. If your child is feeling anxious or vulnerable, focusing on 'passing' or 'failing' can place them under added pressure.

'I feel it's so important not to use the words 'pass' and 'fail'. It's not something anyone can study for. The immune system not being ready for more at a certain point isn't anyone's fault or anything they can affect. I tend to say, 'Great, your body was able to tolerate a bit, which gives us something to build on'. It does help my son to face the next challenge.' – Lynn H

'My daughter, who is ten, said calling it a 'challenge' doesn't always help either as if it doesn't go to plan you feel so negative and like you've personally failed. Language is so important!' – Clare Hussein

4

After diagnosis: the emotional fallout and how to cope in the early days

'Devastated', 'guilty', 'scared', 'lost', 'utterly overwhelmed' – all ways parents have described how they felt when their child was diagnosed with a food allergy.

I remember very well sitting crying in the car on our way home. Our doctor was wonderful – we received all the advice we could possibly need, and a promise to be there to answer any follow-up questions whenever they arose. But it's no under-statement to say it felt completely devastating.

We knew close to nothing about food allergies. I had a friend with a nut allergy but I hadn't, if I'm honest, given it much thought. What was this strange and frightening new world? All of a sudden, food – just food, for goodness' sake – had become a potentially dangerous minefield to be navigated every day. We came away with a ridiculous catalogue of allergies, including wheat, tree nuts, peanuts, sesame, banana ... what on earth was I going to feed him? How would I keep him safe? What about school, parties, sleepovers, first romances, college, work, travel (for perspective, he was barely six months old.).

Other parents describe feeling 'vindicated' and 'relieved' that their concerns are finally taken seriously and found to be justified. Too often mothers – and, yes, it is, sadly, usually mothers – are dismissed as being 'neurotic' or 'over-anxious new parents' when they first try to seek help or insist that their child's symptoms are more than the usual infant complaints:

'I knew something was very wrong and it took us a long time to get that confirmed so, when it was, I was just relieved that my Mum spidey senses were proved right.'

'I felt vindicated and angry that we'd been through so much for it to take nearly 15 months to discover she was allergic ... and yet I'd always been labelled "anxious".'

'Our GP finally believed that I wasn't just a neurotic mother.'

Another common reaction is guilt: 'I felt guilty I hadn't pushed for help sooner'; ' ... guilty because I hadn't recognized anaphylactic reactions for what they were'; 'I felt like it was my fault, that I'd done something to make this happen'; 'I'm atopic so I was responsible'; 'The guilt! What did I eat in pregnancy? What did I not eat? Should I have weaned earlier/later? Should I have/ not have breastfed?'

There is grief, and sadness, for the carefree life they should have had, and for the burden of vigilance and responsibility that they will have to carry from now on. Might they feel different? Left out? Will they be 'excluded from the joy of social eating'?

Parents describe a 'life-changing realization that all was now dangerous'; 'I realized I might lose my baby boy over something as trivial as eating a chocolate bar' or 'I felt scared that simple pleasures, like eating a cupcake, could now pose a risk'. They feel sad at 'the life changes and preventative cautions now needed' and the fact that 'food went from being this thing we never really thought about to being such a big deal – checking packaging, fearing eating out, worrying about leaving her in the charge of others'.

'I felt overwhelmed, it seemed such a big thing to cope with ... and scared about her potentially having a serious and life-threatening reaction ... and sad that this was something that she would have to deal with.'

'I grieved the life I thought she wouldn't be able to lead.'

'It made one of the bits of babyhood I'd most been looking forward to – weaning – so hugely anxiety-ridden.'

That last one was a biggie for us too. The little moments you see other parents share: a Dad in a café tearing off a corner of croissant for his toddler to nibble at; making a normal family meal and then pureeing it for baby to have the following day (something my mum used to do for us); going on holiday and trying new food – seeing the look on their little face as they discover a new taste, a new sensation, instead of reading every look and grimace as the precursor to a possible reaction. It made me feel sad, a little bitter, certainly envious, and there was a sense of loss over what he – and, yes, we – wouldn't experience.

Thoughts race through your head: the things you recall from childhood, which very often centre around food. Pick 'n' mix at the cinema, a towering ice cream sundae from a café at the seaside, a meal at your favourite family restaurant, a grandmother's treasured pudding recipe.

For those of you out there feeling afraid, lost, or wondering where to turn, the message is that you are not alone. The burden of anxiety on the shoulders of families of children with food allergy hasn't gone unnoticed by the experts, either. A 2014 paper by Imperial College found 'increased anxiety and stress' among mothers of food-allergic children compared with mothers of children with no chronic illness.[1]

Food allergy is also associated with a poorer quality of life than other conditions, such as diabetes or asthma, with one review[2] by paediatrician Lars Lange also noting: 'The fear of a child experiencing an allergic reaction is of crucial significance ... Virtually all

---

1 'Anxiety and stress in mothers of food-allergic children', Lau et al, *Paediatric Allergy 7 Immunology*, 2014. See: <https://pubmed.ncbi.nlm.nih.gov/24750570/>

2 'Quality of life in the setting of anaphylaxis and food allergy', L. Lange, *Allergo Journal International*, 2014. See: <https://www.ncbi.nlm.nih.gov/pmc/articles/PMC4479473/>

outdoor activities, such as school events, school trips, overnight stays with friends and parties, are affected. Many children are either excluded from these events or need to be accompanied by their parents until they reach young adulthood. Although parents perceive the resulting overprotectiveness as unbeneficial for their child, they see no alternative.' With time, most parents learn to cope and become more relaxed, the author adds – although new and unfamiliar situations, such as school trips or parties, can bring fear to the fore again. He writes: 'A major cause of parental frustration is the fact that they feel misunderstood by other people and by the public in general. They experience their children being excluded from events or activities, such as sleeping away from home. Parents also often find themselves confronted with family members or carers who question the relevance of their child's food allergy.' However, the paper notes that a 'clear diagnosis with clear recommendations on avoidance can ease the situation for the parents', and recommends doctors adopt a 'calm conversational technique and a realistic assessment of the risks of the disease [which] can be crucial to the family's quality of life for a long period of time'.

The other side of allergies

But ... there are positives, too, that come from diagnosis – assuming your doctor has provided you with all the information and support you need. At the same time as that maelstrom of emotion and worry hits, there's something else rising in you: a determination not to let allergy win.

We are often painted as 'helicopter parents', constantly buzzing around anxiously, unable to let go. But so much of that energy and 'buzziness' goes into creating an environment for our kids where they don't miss out, where anything is possible, where vigilance and practical steps mean they can enjoy the same fun and freedoms as their friends.

'I felt determined not to let them be beaten or weighed down by their allergy, and not be defined by it.'

'It was empowering, because at last we had the knowledge to deal with this.'

We make coping with allergy our mission – finding safe recipes, safe products, advocating on our children's behalf, teaching them how to read labels, ask questions and never eat anything without checking. All of this is not to mollycoddle, but to empower, and free, them. Actually. So tell that to the next busybody who accuses you of being over-protective.

Will I be left to cope on my own now?

The answer to this is, no, you won't. Or you shouldn't. With diagnosis you should be armed with all the information you need to manage this condition.

That means if your child has AAIs, you should have proper training in how to use the device. It means your doctor should direct you to support from other resources – flyers and leaflets from the hospital on managing an avoidance diet; information on the two main charities working with food allergy (Allergy UK and the Anaphylaxis Campaign); access to a dietitian if you feel you need help with recipes and products.

If you need support, don't be afraid to contact your GP or clinic to ask. If you are struggling with meals, ask to speak to a dietitian. If you feel you need extra AAI training, ask to see a nurse. If you are worried about new symptoms, go back to your doctor and talk to them. If you are suffering from anxiety, tell your doctor this, too (see Chapter 17 for more).

Regular follow-ups – ideally annual, if clinics have the capability, or at least every few years – are important to keep track of your child's allergies. Some allergies can be outgrown, or careful reintroduction may sometimes be possible under the guidance of a specialist. You shouldn't be sent away with no hope of a follow-up to come.

The children's allergy department at the Evelina London recommends that, 'at a minimum', children with food allergies should be seen at age four, before they start primary school; age seven to eight in Year 3; age ten to 11 in Year 6; age 12 to 13 in Year 8; and again at 15, in Year 10 to 11. This is 'due to the rate that allergies change and develop'. Families with more complex needs, or multiple allergies, may be seen more frequently. If your child has asthma and a food allergy, they should also be seen in a local asthma clinic at your GP surgery or local hospital.

When your child is around 16, they will be transferred to an adult allergy clinic. Some hospitals now provide a transition clinic for adolescents preparing to move from paediatric to adult care. This is a vulnerable time, so can be hugely beneficial.

Sometimes there is one key piece of advice that stays with you for years to come, and helps to calm you when things seem overwhelming.

For example, when we were reeling from our first diagnosis our allergist told us: 'See the EpiPen as liberating, not limiting'. He didn't mean we could go woo-hoo crazy and ignore advice to avoid our son's allergens. But what I think he meant was, take this and all the information I've given you as a pathway to managing the condition, not a barrier to living life. The more informed we – and our children – are, the better we can cope.

Here are some of the other words of wisdom reported by fellow allergy parents:

'No Epi, no eat'

'Live life, just read the small print!'

'When in doubt, don't eat it.'

'Always pack snacks, so you can be spontaneous.'

'Make plans around people and activities instead of food.'

'Don't be scared to ask if you're unsure. If you need reassurance, ask any question you like. If you don't get it, don't do the activity or eat the food.'

'Necessity is opportunity – we have to create the safe alternatives.'

'Learning to live with severe allergies should mean exactly that: living, as in eating out, going to events, travelling ...'

'Check every label every time – even if it's a product you've bought 100 times over. Ingredients can change.'

'Focus on what you can eat, not what you can't.'

Will my child outgrow their allergies?

This is very often the first question parents ask – is there any hope that my child will grow out of this? Unfortunately, nobody can predict with certainty what the path of your child's allergies will be.

The good news is: generally speaking, the majority of children with food allergy will outgrow it during childhood, especially when it comes to cow's milk, wheat and egg. We discovered that banana allergy is another one that, when it crops up in infancy, is usually outgrown before school age. We were regularly forced to flee toddlers wielding bananas for about two and a half years, before skin prick tests and a hospital food challenge established that he had outgrown that particular one.

On the other hand, allergies to tree nuts, peanuts, sesame, fish and shellfish are less likely to be outgrown. It is also the case that the longer you have an allergy, and the older you are, the more likely it is to stick around. It's important to remember, however, that this is far from definitive – there is always the chance that an allergy may be outgrown, especially as children grow and their bodies change.

A study from the Isle of Wight followed children with peanut allergy for a decade, by which time around ten per cent had outgrown their allergy. It is thought that, by adulthood, around 20 per cent will have outgrown a peanut allergy.

It's precisely because of the possibility of allergies being outgrown that it is important to have a regular review. If you don't have any follow-up appointments booked in, ask your GP to refer you to an allergy clinic.

I've heard people talk about the 'allergic march'. What is it?

The 'allergic march' – also known as the 'atopic march' – refers to the way in which allergic disorders are related. They typically start in the early years in a recognized sequence.

So it usually begins with eczema in babyhood, which, especially if it occurs in the first six months, is associated with the development of food allergy. It is also linked to asthma and hay fever, which tend to start later – around primary school age on average.

But ... while allergy doctors acknowledge the importance of understanding the relationship between these allergic conditions, they increasingly dislike the use of the word 'march', which implies an inevitable progression or worsening. Children's allergy specialist Dr Lauri-Ann Van der Poel says: 'One of the reasons paediatric allergy is one of the most exciting fields in medicine is the explosion in research and knowledge about how to recognize allergic conditions early, treat them more effectively, and to go beyond that to prevent their development.'

So, it does not mean your child's eczema in infancy will automatically progress to the development of asthma in later childhood. Neither does it mean that symptoms will get worse over time. With good allergy advice early on, these various atopic conditions by no means always go hand-in-hand.

Find your community

When we were first diagnosed, more than anything I really, really wanted to find people in the same boat. Nobody else we knew had a child with food allergies. I remember the sheer unbridled joy and excitement when I saw another mum pull out her son's EpiPen pack at a local singing group.

We went to Anaphylaxis Campaign support groups, which I would wholeheartedly recommend. I took to Twitter, Facebook and Instagram, too, and tracked down a lovely community of fellow parents, adults, dietitians, allergy specialists and more (see Resources at the end of this book).

While medical advice should only and always come from your doctor, these platforms have been a lifesaver for the daily practicalities: finding products or recipes, letting off steam about difficulties with school or just having someone there who 'gets it'. There can be a very paternalistic view of social media – that it fuels anxiety and is packed with misinformation. This is, of course, true in some instances, and if you find an online group has your worry levels rising, leave and look elsewhere. But if you find your community, it can provide unparalleled friendship and support.

One thing a doctor can't do is tell you is which Easter eggs are nut allergy-safe this year, which retailers label well for 'may contains' or how to deal with an allergy-sceptic relative.

My point is that you will feel all at sea, bewildered and afraid, but there are plenty sailing on the same choppy waters, so don't be afraid to look for them.

5

Why has my child got food allergies?

It's the question we all ask ourselves – and if we're really lucky (insert sarcasm emoji) it's the question other people ask us too. Did I do something to cause my child's food allergy? Is it somehow my fault?

Simple answer? No, it's categorically not your fault.

The truth is there is no single answer, and currently not enough data to make confident pronouncements – although there are several hypotheses and considerable ongoing research. If anyone tells you they 'know' why food allergies are on the rise, they don't.

Research suggests that the so-called 'allergy epidemic' we are living through may have its roots in events that occurred way back when the parents of children affected were 'in utero', i.e. before birth. This could be a combination of environments and behaviours that we don't yet fully understand. On the other hand, there is emerging evidence that postnatal factors may be associated with increased risk of food allergy.

As Professor Katrina Allen and Dr Jennifer Koplin note in their review 'Prospects for Prevention of Food Allergy',[1] 'there is a rapidly emerging body of research [but] it is not yet clear whether there is one main hypothesis ... a number of factors that act in concert, [or] multiple pathways to the disease'.

Here are some of the main theories and studies:

---

1 'Prospects for Prevention of Food Allergy', Allen et al, *The Journal of Allergy & Clinical Immunology*, 2016. See: <https://pubmed.ncbi.nlm.nih.gov/26755097/>

Sensitization

Generally speaking, a person cannot have an allergic reaction to a substance that he or she has never come across before. So how on earth did my child react to peanut/egg/milk etc. the very first time they encountered it, you may ask? The answer is that their body will have already been exposed to that allergen and become 'sensitized' to it. With children who are at high risk of developing food allergy, this 'sensitization' process means that when the offending allergen is reintroduced to the body, it reacts to it.

The sensitization may have occurred orally – for instance eating egg for the first time with no symptoms, but then reacting the next time – or through the respiratory system (inhaling aeroallergens such as pollen) or via the skin.[2] The mechanisms whereby sensitization leads to allergy are still being explored and are not yet fully understood. But one of the leading theories pinpoints sensitization via broken skin (below).

Dry skin

There is a strong link between eczema and food allergy. Infants with eczema are six times more likely to develop IgE-mediated food allergy[3] and more than half of those with 'moderately severe early onset eczema' – defined as onset before three months and requiring treatment with topical steroids – will develop a proven food allergy by the age of one.

That's us. Our son was five or six weeks old when he began to show signs of eczema, which gradually got more persistent (a red, bumpy, itchy rash across his forehead, cheeks, neck and

---

2 'Mechanisms of food allergy', Sampson et al, *Journal of Allergy & Clinical Immunology*, 2018. See: <https://www.jacionline.org/article/S0091-6749(17)31809-2/pdf>

3 'Prospects for Prevention of Food Allergy', Allen et al, *The Journal of Allergy & Clinical Immunology*, 2016. See: <https://pubmed.ncbi.nlm.nih.gov/26755097/>

torso). The GP struggled to treat it with petroleum creams, hydrocortisone and mild steroids, and antibiotics as it became periodically infected. It probably seems an overreaction to most, but I can't tell you how distressing it was to have a baby with such inflamed and visibly rashy skin. 'Soft as a baby's bottom', 'lovely rosy cheeks', 'peachy' – all those descriptors of infanthood that just didn't tally with our little one.

I remember hearing that Vitamin D might have an effect, and taking him out cosied up against the winter chill to sit on a park bench, face turned to the waning winter sun in the vain hope that it might help. It was hugely upsetting to see his red, scaly skin and wonder why none of the creams were working. Some even seemed to make the flare-ups worse. Plus he smelled variously either of paraffin (the petroleum-based creams) or smelly socks.

We were referred to a dermatologist, who helped us to get the worst of it under control. She explained that finding an emollient that worked was trial and error – you had to keep going until you found the cream that worked for you. She also told us to use steroid cream sparingly as a 'fire-fighting' measure, to dampen down flare-ups as they arose and stop them from spreading. This really worked, and it's a tactic we continue to use today. He doesn't have many flare-ups now but at the first sign we are all over it like a, well, rash. But even as we battled his skin, the notion of food allergy being to blame didn't seriously arise. I remember the skin specialist only once saying, 'The only other thing I can think of is food allergy but you don't even want to go there'. So we didn't. It was only after diagnosis, in conjunction with that strict regime of steroids for flare-ups and twice or thrice daily moisturising cream, that we finally got on top of the outbreaks and he got his baby-soft skin back.

In 2008, professor of paediatric allergy Prof Gideon Lack proposed something he called the 'dual allergen hypothesis'[4] – now dubbed the 'Lack' hypothesis. It suggested that allergic sensitization to foods may occur through exposure to low doses of allergen through the skin, with food allergens absorbed through a damaged skin barrier. And yes, that's us again. How were we to know that sitting with our scaly baby on our lap munching peanut butter on toast or egg mayonnaise sandwiches might be the trigger for what came next?

There is also some suggestion that using creams and lotions containing commonly allergenic ingredients (almond oil was often recommended by midwives back in the day, and some eczema creams even contained peanut oil) may trigger allergies.

The second part of Lack's hypothesis is that oral exposure to these allergens, by eating allergenic food in infancy, may prevent sensitization by promoting oral tolerance and therefore stop the development of the food allergy.

There had been some suggestion that daily moisturising for all babies from birth could reduce the incidence of infantile eczema, too – but the 2020 BEEP (Barrier Enhancement for Eczema Prevention) Study[5] unfortunately found no evidence that this worked. It even showed early signals that daily use of creams may possibly increase the risk of food allergy. This did *not* apply to children already suffering from eczema, for whom the benefit of daily moisturising remains clear (see Chapter 20 for eczema management).

---

4 'Epidemiologic risks for food allergy', G. Lack, *The Journal of Allergy 7 Clinical Immunology*, 2008. See: <https://www.jacionline.org/article/s0091-6749(08)00778-1/fulltext>

5 'Daily emollient during infancy for prevention of eczema: the BEEP randomised controlled trial', Chalmers et al, *The Lancet*, 2020. See: <https://www.thelancet.com/journals/lancet/article/PIIS0140-6736(19)32984-8/fulltext>

Diet and the LEAP study

A 2008 paper by Professor George du Toit et al[6] uncovered something intriguing – a five-fold higher prevalence of peanut allergy in Jewish children in the UK compared to children in Israel. At the time, infants in Israel were commonly weaned on a peanut snack – Bamba – from the age of four to six months. Meanwhile, in the UK at that time (but not now) guidelines recommended avoidance of peanut until after the age of three.

Professor Gideon Lack and colleagues then embarked on what has been dubbed The LEAP Study (Learning Early About Peanut Allergies)[7] – a large trial to assess whether early intro-duction of peanut, between four and 11 months, might protect against peanut allergy in high-risk infants (defined as those with early onset eczema or egg allergy).

Of the children who avoided peanut, 17 per cent developed peanut allergy by the age of five. Yet only three per cent of the children who were randomized to eating the peanut snack developed allergy by the same age. This showed that regular peanut consumption, begun in early infancy and continued until age five, reduced the rate of peanut allergy in at-risk infants by 80 per cent compared to non-peanut consumers.

'For decades allergists have been recommending that young infants avoid consuming allergenic foods such as peanut to prevent food allergies,' noted Professor Lack. 'Our findings suggest that this advice was incorrect and may have contributed to the rise in peanut and other food allergies.'

---

6   'Early consumption of peanuts in infancy is associated with a low prevalence of peanut allergy', Du Toit et al, *The Journal of Allergy & Clinical Immunology*, 2008. See: <https://pubmed.ncbi.nlm.nih.gov/19000582/>

7   Clinical trials investigating how to best prevent Peanut Allergy Lack et al, Immune Tolerance Network. See: <http://www.leapstudy.co.uk>

A subsequent study – LEAP-On[8] – demonstrated that tolerance of peanut persisted in those children even if they stopped eating it. The study followed 556 of the original 640 LEAP children for a one-year period of peanut avoidance. After this time, only 4.8 per cent of the children who had been weaned early on to peanut were found to be allergic. But 18.6 per cent of those that had avoided peanut for the first 11 months of life had a peanut allergy.

The LEAP and LEAP-On participants are now being followed in the LEAP Trio Study, through to the age of 12. The study will also assess their siblings.

The EAT study

The EAT ('Early Introduction of Allergenic Foods to Induce Tolerance') Study[9] was led by the same team, and ran from 2008 to 2015. It looked into when is the best time to introduce allergenic foods into the infant diet to minimize the risk of food allergy developing. The foods investigated were milk, peanut, sesame, fish, egg and wheat.

More than 1,300 mothers and infants were recruited, with half following standard UK advice and asked to exclusively breastfeed for six months before introducing allergenic foods. The other half was asked to introduce the six allergenic foods early – from the age of three months – alongside breastfeeding.

All the children were monitored until three years of age, and the study found that early introduction of allergenic foods may indeed be effective in food allergy prevention. However, it depended on how much of those allergenic foods was

8 'Effect of Avoidance on Peanut Allergy after Early Peanut Consumption', Du Toit et al, *The New England Journal of Medicine*, 2016. See: <https://www.nejm.org/doi/full/10.1056/NEJMoa1514209>

9 'Enquiring About Tolerance (EAT) study: Feasibility of an early allergenic food introduction regimen, Perkin et al, *Journal of Allergy & Clinical Immunology*, 2016. See: <https://www.ncbi.nlm.nih.gov/pmc/articles/PMC4852987/>

consumed: for example optimum weekly consumption was found to be one small boiled egg and 1½ teaspoons of peanut butter. It was also noted that maintaining these amounts was, while safe, not necessarily easy.

The study found:

- Among the infants who consumed the recommended quantity of allergenic foods, there was a two-thirds reduction in overall food allergy.
- There were no cases of peanut allergy among the infants introduced early to peanut, compared to 2.5 per cent among the group that delayed introduction.
- Egg allergy developed in 1.4 per cent of infants who consumed egg early, compared to 5.5 per cent of those that delayed until after six months.
- There were unfortunately no significant effects reported with regards to milk, wheat, sesame or fish.

Further findings, published in 2019, showed that early intro-duction of allergenic foods to 'high-risk' babies significantly reduced the likelihood of developing food allergy. These findings have led to updated advice on weaning children at greater risk of developing food allergies, issued by the British Society of Allergy and Clinical Immunology. See Chapter 6 for details.

Varied diet

There are some suggestions, from European studies, that a diversity of foods introduced in the first year of life may be associated with reduced risk of food allergy and food sensiti-zation. A mix of fresh fruit and vegetables and home-prepared meals may also be in some way preventative. But there need to be bigger studies to determine what the mechanisms might be – improved nutrient levels? Microbial diversity? Higher dietary fibre? The jury is still out. One thing to tell your 'well-meaning' relative: this doesn't mean your baby has allergies because you fed him burgers.

The 'hygiene hypothesis' – then and now

You've probably heard of this one. Too often it's been seized upon to suggest that a child with food allergy has somehow been made to live an overly sanitized, mollycoddled life. Don't even entertain that reading. As with all things allergy, it's way more complicated than that.

In 1989, a landmark paper[10] was published by Dr David Strachan, proposing the 'hygiene hypothesis'. He suggested that the rising incidence of allergic disease was linked to reduced exposure to germs through declining family sizes, less exposure to animals and generally higher standards of cleanliness. He theorized that repeated exposure to microbes at an early age, for example having several siblings, owning a pet or living on a farm, may help our immune systems to adapt and not to overreact to routine environmental stimuli, such as potential allergens. Without this repeated exposure, our developing immune system becomes over-stimulated by harmless substances.

There have been supportive studies since, such as one in Sweden[11] that found children whose parents sucked on their dummy had different oral microbiota and less eczema than children whose parents did not. A secondary analysis of data within the EAT study found living with dogs was associated with a 90 per cent drop in the odds of infants developing food allergy.[12]

---

10 'Hay fever, hygiene, and household size', D. P. Strachan, *The BMJ*, 1989. See: <https://www.ncbi.nlm.nih.gov/pmc/articles/PMC1838109/>

11 'Pacifier cleaning practices and risk of allergy development', Hesselmar et al, *Paediatrics*, 2013. See: <https://pubmed.ncbi.nlm.nih.gov/23650304/>

12 'Dog ownership at three months of age is associated with protection against food allergy', Marrs et al, *European Journal of Allergy & Clinical Immunology*, 2019. See: <https://onlinelibrary.wiley.com/doi/abs/10.1111/all.13868>

A comparison of the prevalence of allergies in the East and West German populations before and after unification seems to back the hypothesis. Before unification, East Germany had more children growing up on farms and in larger families than West Germany, and the population also had much lower rates of allergy and asthma. After unification, when East Germany developed a more western culture, rates of asthma and allergy increased. This effect could not be explained away by increased diagnosis as East Germany had a highly developed healthcare system before unification. And a 2019 study comparing prevalence of child food allergy in rural and urban South Africa also found lower incidence in the rural region.[13]

The 'hygiene hypothesis' has since developed into the 'Old friends mechanism', which emphasizes that the likelihood of developing allergies is related to an individual's microbiome – the population of microbes living in and on the human body.[14] Exposure in early life to a diversity of microbes, which have evolved alongside humans for millions of years, helps to develop a properly regulated immune system that does not overreact to harmless allergens. Changes to human lifestyles, including less breastfeeding, smaller family size and increased antibiotic use, have affected exposure to these microbes. In a more 'hygienic' environment, the immune system has less need to fight against as many invading microbes and so its responses are 'skewed'.

Some have suggested 'biome depletion' as a better term than 'hygiene hypothesis'. The theory has often been misinterpreted to mean people are too clean, or not exposed enough to infectious diseases. Research is ongoing to find out more about the

---

13 'Rural and urban food allergy prevalence in from the South African Food Allergy study', Botha et al, *Journal of Allergy & Clinical Immunology*, 2019. See: <https://www.jacionline.org/article/S0091-6749(18)31130-8/abstract>

14 'Allergy: Policy Briefing', *British Society for Immunology*, 2017. See: <https://www.immunology.org/sites/default/files/Allergy%20briefing.pdf>

links between factors such as family size, pet ownership and living on a farm, and lower incidence of allergy.

Other theories

Over the years you are cast iron guaranteed to come across countless news reports declaring the discovery of new 'causes' of food allergy. Some you will shrug off, others will niggle away at the back of your head: I exercised and swam regularly when pregnant with my son, and three years into our allergy journey was faced with the calamitous headline 'MOTHERS WHO SWIM DURING PREGNANCY INCREASE THEIR CHILD'S RISK OF ECZEMA AND ASTHMA'.[15]

Studies have also hypothesized links between C-sections and allergy, and between antibiotics and allergy. And, yes, both my children were born via emergency C-section and antibiotics were involved. But one is allergic, one is not. And, either way, they possibly wouldn't be here at all without the C-sections.

It's worth drilling into the detail of the studies to get some perspective. In 2019, the Baby Biome study reported that babies born by C-section had different gut bacteria to those born vaginally.[16] However, it also found that, after weaning, these levels of microbiome had largely levelled out. Further study is needed to establish whether these early differences in gut microbiome lead to any health issues, such as allergy. Researchers also emphasized that C-sections are often a life-saving procedure and the right choice for many women and babies.

---

15 'Mothers who swim during pregnancy increase their child's risk of eczema and asthma, scientists warn', *Daily Mail*, 2013. See: <https://www.dailymail.co.uk/news/article-2408374/Mothers-swimpregnancy-increase-childs-risk-eczema-asthma-scientists-warn.html>

16 'Stunted microbiota and opportunistic pathogen colonisation in caesarean-section birth', Shao et al, *Nature*, 2019. See: <https://www.nature.com/articles/s41586-019-1560-1>

Another hypothesis is that the use of antibiotics in infancy may have some link to allergic disease, but studies have not established a causal relationship. It may be that infants already at increased risk of developing allergic disease are more susceptible to bacterial infections requiring antibiotics. Of course, experts caution against overuse of antibiotics when not needed – for example for a virus or a cold – but children should absolutely have antibiotics they have been prescribed to treat infection.

Meanwhile, that pregnant mothers swimming story? Researchers from the St John's Institute of Dermatology and University of Manchester reviewed existing evidence to find 'exposure to certain airborne chemicals during pregnancy and in early life may play a contributory role in influencing suscep-tibility to atopic allergy'.[17] Chlorine, cleaning products and cosmetics may all be implicated ... or may not.

As lead researcher Dr John McFadden noted:[18] 'We in the science world are still struggling to find the exact cause of this rise [in atopic disease]. Several theories have been put out there ... We have now postulated another possibility. We have not proved anything, we are not saying this is the cause, this is a hypothesis but we do know we are using far more chemicals than we did 50 years ago, whether it is in personal care products or processed food, and we think this should be looked at and studied more.'

The fact is, the physical and mental benefits to me – and probably my son – of my having swam regularly while pregnant dramatically outweigh any not (yet) proven links to whether he did or did not develop allergies.

---

17 'The hapten-atopy hypothesis III: the potential role of airborne chemicals', McFadden et al, *British Journal of Dermatology*, 2013. See: <https://onlinelibrary.wiley.com/doi/abs/10.1111/bjd.12602>

18 'Expectant mothers who swim 'may give baby asthma', *The Telegraph*, 2013. See: <https://www.telegraph.co.uk/news/health/news/10278263/Expectantmothers-who-swim-may-give-baby-asthma.html>

Whatever you may read, and whatever new studies throw up, please don't berate yourself for things you did, or didn't do, when pregnant, breastfeeding and beyond. I mean, other studies suggest children whose grandmother smoked may have double the risk of developing childhood asthma.[19] What are you going to do with that information? All this research is vital and will feed into future increased knowledge and understanding. But when it comes to you, and your child now, it's truly not worth lingering on.

---

19 'Grandmothers' Smoking Linked To Grandchildren's Asthma Decades Later', *Science Daily*, 2005. See: <https://www.sciencedaily.com/releases/2005/05/050505224059.htm>

6

Pregnancy, siblings and weaning

Aside from a panic at four weeks when she developed a horrid eczema-type rash across her face and neck (which disappeared three fraught weeks later) our youngest daughter has remained, dare I say it, food allergy free. But I won't say the journey through pregnancy and weaning has been without its stresses. When we first considered a baby number two, among the first questions on my mind were – how likely is this little one to develop allergies? And is there anything I can do to stop it?

Reassuringly, the likelihood of a second child also being food allergic isn't as high as you might think. Recent studies have shown less than 14 per cent of siblings of food allergic children had food allergies too.[1]

Our son's allergy doctor said eczema in early infancy would be a suggestive sign, so if the new baby were to develop the same rashy skin as her brother, he would book us in for an appointment to get her checked out. At the time – more than eight years ago – a small number of trials had also looked into the efficacy of taking probiotics to prevent atopic disease. There was some suggestion that probiotics given to the mother before delivery and during breastfeeding might confer protection from atopic eczema for the infant. In theory, it made sense, fitting in with the notion that low diversity of microbes in the gut is strongly linked with allergy and asthma. Supplementing with 'good bacteria' might seem a promising tactic. Our doctor said the jury was out, but that it couldn't hurt. The studies focused

1 'Food Allergy Sensitization and Presentation in Siblings of Food Allergic Children', Gupta et al, *Journal of Allergy & Clinical Immunology*, 2016. See: <https://www.ncbi.nlm.nih.gov/pmc/articles/PMC5010481/>

on a specific strain called Lactobacillus rhamnosus GG, so I tracked down a stash and popped a capsule a day through pregnancy and, after my daughter was born, for the first three months of breastfeeding.

In the end, the excitement around probiotics – which, to be fair, remained mixed with scepticism – has subsided somewhat. There is still no evidence to suggest taking probiotics can prevent food allergy in infants. Specialist allergy dietitian Carina Venter says: 'The only association between Lactobacillus GG supplementation in pregnancy, lactation and early life is reduced odds of developing eczema, but the evidence is not strong enough to recommend routine supplementation.'

But is there anything else that can help? Here's the lowdown on the latest thinking around pregnancy, weaning and beyond …

How likely is a sibling to develop food allergies too?

A 2016 study (Gupta et al)[2] published in the *Journal of Allergy & Clinical Immunology* found that only 13.6 per cent of siblings of children with food allergy also had a food allergy themselves.

This means the risk is actually only minimally higher than in the general population. A greater proportion of siblings may show sensitization to certain allergens, through testing, but don't experience any food allergy symptoms when they eat those foods and so are not allergic. The same study found that only one in ten siblings of children with a specific food allergy end up being allergic to the same thing.

---

2 'Food Allergy Sensitization and Presentation in Siblings of Food Allergic Children', Gupta et al, *Journal of Allergy & Clinical Immunology*, 2016. See: <https://www.ncbi.nlm.nih.gov/pmc/articles/PMC5010481/>

Should I avoid any foods while pregnant?

No. In the past, women were advised to avoid peanuts during pregnancy. However this guidance has now been changed as avoidance of commonly allergenic foods has not been shown to play any part in preventing food allergy in infants.

What can I do in pregnancy to lower the risk of my child having allergies?

It's boring but … official advice is that a balanced, healthy diet with lots of vegetables and fibre can only be a good thing.

The BSACI guidance, *'Preventing food allergy in your baby'*,[3] also suggests that Omega-3 fatty acids, found in oily fish such as salmon, trout, mackerel and fresh (not canned) tuna 'may help reduce the risk of eczema and allergic sensitization in early life'. Pregnant women should eat no more than two portions of oily fish per week.

If you are vegetarian or vegan, it is harder to find the long-chain Omega 3 fats such as DHA found in oily fish, but short-chain Omega 3, such as ALA, can be found in flax and chia seeds, walnuts, rapeseed and soybean oil, and soya beans. DHA can also be found in algae-based supplements such as softgels and oils (but you will need to check these are suitable for pregnancy, and don't contain Vitamin A).

They also advise following general guidelines to take folic acid and Vitamin D supplements during pregnancy (again, there's no current evidence that Vitamin D can prevent allergy but it's an important supplement regardless).

---

3 'Preventing food allergy in your baby: A summary for parents', BSACI. See: <https://www.bsaci.org/wp-content/uploads/2020/02/pdf_Infant-feedingand-allergy-prevention-PARENTS-FINAL-booklet.pdf>

A 2021 paper by Venter et al[4] found that eating more vegetables and yoghurt, and fewer sugary, fatty and low fibre foods, may be protective against allergic conditions including rhinitis, eczema and asthma. One theory behind vegetables and yoghurt being potentially beneficial is that they have been reported to increase gut microbiome diversity. The study also reported that cutting down your intake of red meat, cold sugar-sweetened cereal, fried potatoes, and 100 per cent pure fruit juice may be associated with a lower prevalence of eczema, wheeze, asthma and rhinitis. However the study did not show association between maternal diet and food allergy, and further trials are needed to establish whether the findings bear out.

Does breastfeeding stop allergies?

Again, no, there is no evidence to suggest that breastfeeding prevents allergies – but it is recommended for the first six months of life, when possible, because it confers other health benefits. If breastfeeding isn't available, the BSACI recommends use of a standard cow's milk formula rather than any 'low-allergy' formula – unless, of course, the baby is allergic to milk.

What is the current advice on weaning?

Current UK government advice is to introduce common allergens such as milk, eggs, peanut, tree nut, wheat, soya, fish and seeds from six months of age, and in small amounts. But, as covered in Chapter 5, studies now show that delaying the introduction of commonly allergenic foods, such as egg and peanut, to siblings of children with food allergies may actually increase risk. And there may be particular benefit in introducing

4 'The maternal diet index in pregnancy is associated with offspring allergic diseases: the Healthy Start study', Venter et al, *Allergy*, 2021. See: <https://pubmed.ncbi.nlm.nih.gov/34018205/>

these foods from four months of age in children at higher risk of developing food allergy. Allergy experts hope that as evidence grows, general guidelines will be revised and updated.

In 2018, the British Society of Allergy and Immunology (BSACI) published guidance in association with the Food Allergy Specialist Group of the British Dietetic Association, which paves the way for future changes. *Preventing Food Allergy in Your Baby* advises healthcare professionals and families of so-called 'high-risk' infants on how to implement available evidence from the LEAP and EAT studies (see Chapter 5) on early introduction of commonly allergenic foods.

High-risk infants are those with eczema (particularly if it is very bad or began in the first three months of life) or those who already have a food allergy.

So how do I wean a 'high-risk' baby?

The BSACI guidelines state: 'In babies at higher risk of developing food allergy, studies have shown that starting egg and peanut earlier – from four months of age – can help prevent allergy to [those foods].' They also recommend introducing other common allergens, if they are part of your family's diet, before the age of one.

The first thing to remember, of course, is that you should never give your child food he or she is already allergic to. If your baby has troublesome eczema or an existing allergy, then have a conversation with your doctor about your plans to wean early, so they can give you all the information you need.

You can also see the BSACI summary guidelines here <https://www.bsaci.org/wp-content/uploads/2020/02/pdf_Infant-feeding-and-allergy-prevention-PARENT-SUMMARY-FINAL.pdf> and visit <https://www.bsaci.org/wp-content/uploads/2020/02/pdf_Infant-feeding-and-allergy-prevention-PARENTS-FINAL-booklet.pdf> for further detail.

Preventing food allergy in your baby:
A summary for parents

Current advice from the UK health departments for healthy babies is:

- Exclusive breastfeeding for around the first 6 months of life.
- From around 6 months of age (but not before 4 months), introduce complementary foods (solids)
  – including foods known to cause food allergies – alongside continued breastfeeding.
- Excluding egg and peanut from your baby's diet may increase their risk of food allergy.

- **When your baby is ready, at around 6 months of age, you can start to feed them complementary foods** (solids) – usually as pureed foods. Start by offering small amounts of vegetables, fruit, starchy foods, protein, pasteurised dairy. Never add salt or sugar - they don't need it.
- In addition to fruit and vegetables, include foods that are part of your family's normal diet which are commonly associated with food allergies. *If this includes egg and peanut, aim to introduce these by one year of age, and continue to feed these to your baby as part of their usual diet.*

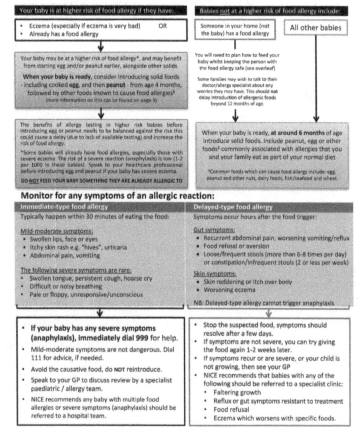

Your baby is at higher risk of food allergy if they have:	**Babies not at a higher risk of food allergy include:**
• Eczema (especially if eczema is very bad) OR • Already has a food allergy	Someone in your home (not the baby) has a food allergy All other babies

Your baby may be at a higher risk of food allergy*, and may benefit from starting egg and/or peanut earlier, alongside other solids.

When your baby is ready, consider introducing solid foods - including cooked egg, and then **peanut** - from age 4 months, followed by other foods known to cause food allergies§ *(more information on this can be found on page 9)*

The benefits of allergy testing in higher risk babies before introducing egg or peanut needs to be balanced against the risk this could cause a delay (due to lack of available testing) and increase the risk of food allergy.

*Some babies will already have food allergies, especially those with severe eczema. The risk of a severe reaction (anaphylaxis) is low (1-2 per 1000 in these babies). Speak to your healthcare professional before introducing egg and peanut if your baby has severe eczema.

DO **NOT** FEED YOUR BABY SOMETHING THEY ARE ALREADY ALLERGIC TO

You will need to plan how to feed your baby whilst keeping the person with the food allergy safe (see overleaf)

Some families may wish to talk to their doctor/allergy specialist about any worries they may have. This should **not** delay introduction of allergenic foods beyond 12 months of age.

When your baby is ready, **at around 6 months** of age introduce solid foods. Include peanut, egg or other foods§ commonly associated with allergies that you and your family eat as part of your normal diet

§Common foods which can cause food allergy include: egg, peanut and other nuts, dairy foods, fish/seafood and wheat.

Monitor for any symptoms of an allergic reaction:

Immediate-type food allergy	**Delayed-type food allergy**
Typically happen within 30 minutes of eating the food:	Symptoms occur hours after the food trigger:
Mild-moderate symptoms: • Swollen lips, face or eyes • Itchy skin rash e.g. "hives", urticaria • Abdominal pain, vomiting	Gut symptoms: • Recurrent abdominal pain, worsening vomiting/reflux • Food refusal or aversion • Loose/frequent stools (more than 6-8 times per day) or constipation/infrequent stools (2 or less per week)
The following severe symptoms are rare: • Swollen tongue, persistent cough, hoarse cry • Difficult or noisy breathing • Pale or floppy, unresponsive/unconscious	Skin symptoms: • Skin reddening or itch over body • Worsening eczema NB: Delayed-type allergy cannot trigger anaphylaxis

• If your baby has any **severe symptoms (anaphylaxis), immediately dial 999** for help.
 • Mild-moderate symptoms are not dangerous. Dial 111 for advice, if needed.
 • Avoid the causative food, do **NOT** reintroduce.
 • Speak to your GP to discuss review by a specialist paediatric / allergy team.
 • NICE recommends any baby with multiple food allergies or severe symptoms (anaphylaxis) should be referred to a hospital team.
	• Stop the suspected food, symptoms should resolve after a few days.
	 • If symptoms are not severe, you can try giving the food again 1-2 weeks later.
	 • If symptoms recur or are severe, or your child is not growing, then see your GP
	 • NICE recommends that babies with any of the following should be referred to a specialist clinic:
	    • Faltering growth
	    • Reflux or gut symptoms resistant to treatment
	    • Food refusal
	    • Eczema which worsens with specific foods.

Used with permission from the BSACI

Once you have talked it over with your doctor, ensure that your baby is developmentally ready for weaning – this means that they should be able to sit up unaided in a high chair and hold their neck and head steady, and are able to swallow foods (they don't 'push' out more with their tongue than they take in).

When introducing peanuts or tree nuts, these should never be given to babies or very young children whole, or coarsely chopped. Globs of nut butter should also be avoided, too, as these all pose serious choking risks. Instead, use 1 teaspoon of smooth peanut butter mixed with 1 tablespoon of warm, pre-boiled water or baby's usual milk. This can be mixed with a fruit or vegetable puree for taste. If age appropriate, 'puffed' peanut snacks (e.g. Bamba) may be used, or peanuts ground to a fine powder and mixed into baby porridge or purees.

Only introduce one allergenic food at a time and start low – for example with just ¼ of a teaspoon, increasing slowly over a number of days. Build up to 2 level teaspoons of peanut or tree nuts per week and, once successfully introduced, try to feed them to your baby at least once a week.

If you are introducing eggs, use in-date British Lion-stamped eggs and offer them scrambled, soft or hard-boiled, or in an omelette. You could also mash cooked egg into baby rice or pureed vegetables. Aim to introduce at least one egg over the course of a week. When introducing wheat, try soft pasta shapes, Weetabix, toast fingers or couscous. Sesame can be introduced as hummus, or you could add crushed seeds to yoghurt or fruit purees. Introduce pasteurized cow's milk as yoghurt, or add whole milk to mashed potato and sauces.

In an ideal world, and with all the resources to hand, high-risk infants might be allergy tested first – or at least parents may prefer this. I know we did. But, in reality, if allergy testing is not locally available, or there is a long wait, this needs to be weighed against the risks that delaying introduction may increase the risk of developing a food allergy. It's a fine balance, and one that the BSACI advises parents of 'high-risk' children to discuss with their healthcare providers first. You also need to be aware that there is a possibility your baby will have an allergic reaction.

In a paper accompanying the new guidelines, the authors note: 'Healthcare professionals should help parents to make an informed decision ... This will depend on their under-standing of the potential for an allergic reaction when allergenic foods are introduced ... and the availability of allergy testing within the local clinical service ... This is a pragmatic decision, based not only on the current availability of allergy testing ... but also on the basis that, to date, no life-threatening reactions have been reported in infants related to the introduction of allergenic foods.' They add: '[S]creening is not generally offered in those countries where peanut is introduced in infancy, and this has not caused major public health concerns.'

Specialist allergy dietitian Carina Venter is encouraging about early introduction of allergenic foods: 'The group with eczema is particularly the group that should start early! It is a race against time. I say to families: "Let's get the allergen into the gut (the friendly immune system) before it penetrates the skin (the unfriendly immune system)".'

Allergy UK notes in its online guide, *Weaning Your Food Allergic Baby:* '[T]o help put your mind at ease, it is estimated that 998-999 out of 1000 babies will NOT have a severe reaction. Also, reassuringly, no life-threatening reactions have been reported as a result of early introduction of allergenic foods in an infant's diet.'

If you decide not to introduce allergenic foods early, try to introduce egg, peanut and other common allergens to your baby by 12 months and, if no reactions occur, keep them in their diet regularly.

General weaning tips

If your baby already has allergies, introducing any new foods – not only the commonly allergenic ones – can be a highly stressful time. It's a little bit devastating too, honestly, when you see friends happily doling out little bits of this and that at random and enjoying watching their babies experience the delight (and disgust) of the new.

If you are just trying to get some more new things into your allergic child's diet, it's a good idea to:

- Keep a food diary, making note of what you introduce and when, so you can monitor potential reactions.
- Introduce new foods every three days or so, so you can isolate anything that may be causing an issue.
- Introduce new food when your baby is well, and you have time to observe them afterwards.
- If you are nervous, you could start with a tiny amount, then wait 20 minutes to observe for any symptoms, before giving a little more and building up to a small portion size. Or even build up over the course of a week.
- Once you have introduced a new food safely, try to keep it in your child's diet regularly.
- Prioritize the foods that are central to your own family's diet. This is simply about making life easier for you as a family.
- If you think your child is displaying any allergic symptoms, stop giving them the food and seek advice from a doctor.

How do I keep allergenic food in my non-allergic child's diet?

Once you're past the weaning stage, it becomes a bit of a logistical challenge to keep the foods one child is allergic to in another child's diet. Among all the well-intentioned advice to introduce egg, peanut and so on as early as possible – and keep it regular – the practicalities are often overlooked. It's not simply a fear that younger siblings may also be allergic; it's also the knowledge that babies and kids have really shitty table manners.

If I'd given our toddler daughter a peanut butter sandwich she'd have used it as a hat and then trundled off to bite her brother. So, while the research shows we'd be better off allowing our non-allergic younger kids to eat everything their elder siblings are allergic to, the reality isn't as straightforward as that.

What was the answer? Send our baby daughter off overnight to the grandparents? Well, at 21 months she was still waking up all hours of the night screaming for boob. Do it while her brother was at nursery? He was only in nursery two mornings a week and they ate all of their meals together.

In the end, I took to taking her for scrambled egg lunches once a week while my husband stayed home with her brother. That first time, it was a very odd feeling. I had (have) never been able to walk off the street into a restaurant, sit down and order anything on a whim for my son. It was nice. I felt guilty, too, about dining out with his sister, so I bought him a T-shirt with a robot on.

Despite an infuriatingly slow start (ignoring the egg, concentrating on the toast) she ended up wolfing down a fair bit. As predicted, we had egg in her ears, up the sleeves of her jumper, on my leg and all over the floor. So we went to the café loo to scrub down. Back home, it was straight to the bathroom for a strip, clothes bundled into the washing machine, hands and face washed with soap and water, teeth brushed, toothbrush slooshed twice (she had a fancy for ramming it into her brother's mouth when he wasn't looking) and into some clean new togs. Job done. Until the next time.

I have to confess we've veered off the path fairly regularly – time, work, school, pandemics, have all conspired to make it difficult to carve out a little free time to take one child off for an elaborate allergy-packed banquet. When she was at nursery, they would often give the kids hummus, so that ticked one off the list. When she was younger, we'd keep a jar of peanut butter in a plastic bag in a top cupboard, along with a stash of disposable spoons and a spare toothbrush. The spoon went in the bin after she had her dose, and we gave her teeth a brush with the secret toothbrush and popped it back up in the cupboard until the next time.

Now, she gets the odd contraband fix at friends' houses or the occasional peanut butter cookie when her brother is elsewhere. It's probably not optimum management but it's as much as we can do.

If you're giving allergens at home, these tips may help:

- Lay wipe-clean matting on the floor beneath your child's chair.
- Limit the feeding to one spot – a high-chair or the kitchen table.
- Invest in a roll-up washable place mat.
- Keep plenty of wipes or washable cloths to hand to give your child a going over afterwards.
- Clean face and hands and make sure there's no food in their hair or dropped on the floor.
- Wash utensils and surfaces with warm, soapy water and put the sponge or cloth in the washing machine.
- If it's been a messy meal, throw those clothes straight into the washing machine and swap for a clean set.

Should I avoid foods my child is allergic to while breastfeeding?

Five or ten years ago, breastfeeding mothers may routinely have been told to remove their child's allergens from their own diet, too. But, increasingly, studies suggest that the quantities of allergen in breastmilk are so low as to be highly unlikely to cause a reaction. One 2020 paper[5] found that, for more than 99 per cent of infants with proven cow's milk allergy, the breastmilk of a cow's milk-consuming woman 'contains insufficient milk allergen to trigger an allergic reaction'. The paper also posits that advice to swap breastfeeding for formula is often directly supported by formula companies.

Anecdotally, many mothers do notice a link between their child's eczema, or even other symptoms, and their consumption of certain foods. However, this may in part be due to accidental exposure – for example, the food coming into contact with the child in other ways.

That's not to dismiss parents' concerns. Our own allergy doctor believes the impetus should come from the mother: if she sees a response in her baby and wants to eliminate a certain food for that reason, then that should be her decision, rather than one imposed as a general rule by a doctor or dietitian.

---

5   Assessment of Evidence About Common Infant Symptoms and Cow's Milk Allergy', Munblit et al, *JAMA Paediatrics*, 2020. See: https://jamanetwork.com/journals/jamapediatrics/article-abstract/2764081

7

Busting some myths and misconceptions

Why your grandma didn't have food allergies

... (and no, it isn't because we're faking them now.)

One of the most common – and tiresome – tropes wheeled out by detractors as 'proof' that allergies don't really exist and are a figment of our pampered minds is the statement: 'Well, allergies didn't exist in my/my grandparent's/Ethelred the Unready's day.'

They (probably) did. The first account of food allergy is generally attributed to Hippocrates (460–377 BC), who referred to the presence of 'hostile humors' (hi IgE antibodies!) in some men that made them 'suffer badly' after eating cheese. Then there's a poem by Roman philosopher Titus Lucretius Cato (98–55 BC) that features the line, 'What is food to one, to another is rank poison.'[1] A little further along the line, rumour has it that King Richard III developed hives and an itchy mouth after eating strawberries.[2]

Then there's the other fact – which is that, sadly, since 1990 the incidence of food allergy has, indeed, escalated into what

---

1 'Food Allergy: Past, present and future', H. Sampson, *Allergology International*, 2016. See: <https://www.sciencedirect.com/science/article/pii/S1323893016301137>

2 'Was the downfall of Richard III caused by a strawberry?', *New Statesman*, 2013. <https://www.newstatesman.com/ideas/2013/08/was-downfall-richardiii-caused-strawberry>

some describe as an epidemic. Allergy is now the most common chronic disease in childhood.

So, yes, there wasn't as much incidence of food allergy in your grandma's day, but that's not because we're making it up.

'If you think in terms of decades, are we seeing more food allergy now than we were 20 or 30 years ago? I think we can confidently say yes,' paediatric allergy consultant Professor Adam Fox told *The Guardian* in 2018. 'If you look at the research from the 1990s and early 2000s there is pretty good data that the amount of peanut allergy trebled in a very short period.'

Seven times as many people were admitted to hospital with severe allergic reactions in Europe in 2015 than in 2005. In the 20 years to 2012, there was a 615 per cent increase in the rate of hospital admissions for anaphylaxis in the UK, and the percentage of children diagnosed with allergic rhinitis and eczema have both trebled over the last 30 years.[3]

The myths and misconceptions

Each reaction will be worse than the last

You cannot predict the future severity of an allergic reaction – and this goes both ways. While a previously mild reaction does not guarantee any subsequent reactions will follow the same path, it is not the case that reactions automatically increase in severity with each exposure.

There are many factors that come into play to trigger an allergic reaction, alongside the allergen itself – such as how much food has been eaten, what form that food takes, whether the person is unwell or stressed, has consumed alcohol, or has just been exercising vigorously.

---

3 'Sense About Science: Making Sense of Allergies', 2015. See: <https://senseaboutscience.org/wp-content/uploads/2016/09/Making-Sense-of-Allergies-1.pdf>

The results of IgE tests can also not be used to predict severity. There are new modes of testing afoot (see Chapter 22) which may, in the future, allow more accurate predictions. For now, it is the case that food allergy can be unpredictable.

Vaccines cause allergies

There have been several large studies investigating the relationship between vaccines and allergies. Large cohort studies in the USA, Sweden and Australia found no association between the receipt of childhood vaccines and atopic conditions including asthma, eczema, food allergy and hay fever.

A German study compared pre-unification East Germany, when vaccination was compulsory and therefore at close to 100 per cent, with post-unification Germany, when immunization rates decreased. Prior to reunification there were hardly any allergies, after reunification allergies became more common.[4]

Children with egg allergy can't have the MMR or flu vaccines

There is an enduring misconception that children with egg allergy cannot have the MMR or flu vaccines. For the MMR jab, egg allergy – however severe – is not a contraindication and there is no increased risk. And the so-called 'SNIFFLE' studies[5] (which our son took part in) have confirmed that the 'nasal spray' (Fluenz Tetra) versions of the flu vaccine are safe in egg-allergic children, including those with previous anaphylaxis. The only exception is those with life-threatening reactions to egg who have required intensive care, and this is because there is little data given such reactions are 'vanishingly rare'.

---

4 'Do immunisations cause allergies?' *Vaccines Today*, 2020. See: <https://www.vaccinestoday.eu/faq/do-immunisations-cause-allergies/>

5 'Safety of live attenuated influenza vaccine in yoiung people with egg allergy: multicentre prospective cohort study', Turner et al, *BMJ*, 2015. See: <https://www.bmj.com/content/351/bmj.h6291>

There are also no-egg and low-egg versions of the injectable flu vaccine that can be safely given. The Green Book[6] of immunization used by doctors details this, and also that the vaccines may be used in primary care and – in the case of the nasal spray – in schools, with the normal precautions taken.

The Green Book is updated every year and is available online at gov.uk.

Junk food causes allergies

'JUNK FOOD MAY BE FUELLING RISE IN FOOD ALLERGIES, SAY EXPERTS'[7]

Headlines like this are the bane of food allergy families' lives. In 2019 a very small Italian study – involving just 23 children with food allergies – suggested there were raised levels of substances called AGEs (glycation end products) in children with food allergies.

AGEs occur naturally in the body, but are found in high levels in processed foods and cooked meats and have been linked to conditions including diabetes. Researchers claimed the children with food allergies in their study ate 20–40 per cent more junk food than the allergy-free peers. However, allergy experts have said the research was too small to take into account other possible factors and there was no evidence to say junk food 'caused' food allergies.

Not letting your kid eat mud caused their allergies

This is a flipping around of the 'hygiene hypothesis' (see Chapter 5). But it's not true or fair to extrapolate a population-wide theory to individuals. Yes, we live in a cleaner, more hygienic

---

6 'Immunisation against infectious disease: the Green Book'. See: <https://www.gov.uk/government/collections/immunisation-against-infectious-disease-the-green-book#the-green-book>

7 'Junk food may be fuelling rise in food allergies, say experts'. *The Guardian*, 2019. See: <https://www.theguardian.com/society/2019/jun/08/junk-food-rise-food-allergies-children>

environment where all of us are exposed to fewer microbiomes. It doesn't mean you, or that parent over there, caused your son's food allergies by not letting him eat dirt.

A little won't hurt

For someone with a food allergy, even a tiny amount of a food allergen can cause a severe reaction. You must remove the allergen completely from your diet to stay well and safe, which usually – unless your doctor specifically advises otherwise – includes avoiding cross contamination (that means tiny amounts of the food you are allergic to contaminating the food you are eating).

Peanut is the most dangerous food allergy

Peanut has acquired a reputation as the bad boy on the block and, while it can be the culprit in many severe reactions, it isn't alone. Virtually any food can cause an allergic reaction.

In fact, an Imperial College London study found that more severe allergic reactions among children in the UK are caused by milk than by peanut.[8] Lead author Dr Paul Turner said: 'There is now a lot of awareness of allergies to peanut and tree nut, but many people think milk allergy is mild, perhaps because most children outgrow it. However, for those who don't, it remains a big problem because milk is so common in our diet, and people don't realize how dangerous it can be.'

All allergic reactions are the same

It would be so handy if they were ... but sadly they aren't. As mentioned previously, allergies are not 'one size fits all'. Not only can reactions differ, but people can differ in their reactions, and reactions can differ depending on the food.

For example, egg allergy might present with tummy ache, or

---

8 'Food anaphylaxis in the United Kingdom: analysis of national data, 1998-2018'. Conrado et al, *BMJ*, 2021. See: <https://www.bmj.com/content/372/bmj.n733>

peanut allergy with itchy eyes and sneezing. There's a misconception too that an anaphylactic reaction always includes hives, whereas they are, in fact, absent in around ten per cent of anaphylaxis cases. The key thing is to learn about the various signs and symptoms and make sure you, your child and anyone who cares for him or her is equally well-versed.

I can cure your allergies

There's a whole industry that has sprung up to exploit people's anxiety and confusion, claiming to offer high street or DIY tests for food allergy (kinesiology, cytotoxic testing, hair testing, Vega testing, IgG or intolerance testing ... see Chapter 3).

Similarly, there's an industry that has arisen around claims to treat allergies. These include NAET, or Nambudripad's Allergy Elimination Techniques. It's based on the idea that allergies are caused by 'energy blockage', which can be diagnosed by muscle testing and then cured by acupuncture. There is zero evidence to support these claims.

The only genuine tests are skin prick tests and blood tests for IgE allergy (see Chapter 3), which should only ever be used in a clinical setting (not at home or on the high street) and analysed by a doctor.

There is a considerable amount of genuine research ongoing into treatments and cures for allergy – things like immunotherapy, for instance – of which more in Chapter 22. But as for the 'alternative' and high street offerings – don't waste your money.

The silly things they say

Entry into 'Life With a Food-Allergic Kid' territory brings with it the boundless joy of people offering unhelpful advice. I'm not sure why it is that a food allergy diagnosis sparks a stream of unsolicited opinions but, well, it does. Brace yourself. Some are well-meaning, but ill-advised, others outright rude and the rest just really stupid.

Here's a handy Top 12 compiled from my own experience and other parents who kindly shared ...

1 'Ooh *excitedly* has he had one of those anaphylactic thingies yet?'
2 'It must be because you're vegetarian.'
3 Nurse: 'How much does your baby's allergy affect your choice of days out and holidays?' Me (shellshocked mum to newly-diagnosed six-month-old): 'Not much, really.' Nurse: 'Oh, but it *will* ...'
4 'Gosh, what on earth CAN he eat?'
5 'Aren't you brave taking him out?'
6 'Oh, he doesn't *look* ill.'
7 'I heard it's because of all the processed food people eat.'
8 'Just pick the nuts off that and you'll be fine.'
9 'Oh my god, I couldn't live like that.'
10 'Just try a bit and see what happens.'
11 'Don't worry about it – you've got the EpiPen if you need it.'
12 'Ah, they'll grow out of it.'

8

Shopping for your food allergic child

Those first few days and weeks following diagnosis are nerve-wracking, confusing and filled to the brim with anxiety. You're let loose clutching an encyclopaedic list of foods to avoid and every social situation, every celebration, every trip, seems fraught with danger.

You should have been given at least a leaflet of foods and their derivatives to watch out for, and hopefully some safe product recommendations and recipes to fill those sudden gaps. Your GP or allergy specialist can refer you to a dietitian to provide these things, if you find yourself struggling.

Before we faced food allergies we blithely thought that having a nut allergy just meant, well, not eating those actual nuts, duh. But it's all so much more complicated than that. You have to navigate the minefield of allergen labelling – what does 'may contain?' mean? Is soya lecithin OK if I have a soya allergy? How much egg is too much egg if my child can tolerate it baked but not raw? How do I find a birthday cake for my egg, nut and wheat-free toddler? Why does everything on the super-market shelves say the equivalent of 'may contain all allergens that ever existed and more'?

I've definitely cried in the supermarket, more than once. And, yes, sometimes I take out my rage on unsafe packets of food with an extra squeeze or a surreptitious punch. (I admitted to this on Twitter once, and it transpires I'm not alone. Obviously I am not inciting you to squeeze biscuits. But sometimes it helps.)

Not only does every meal you cook become a minefield of label checking and anxiously staring at your child's face to make sure he or she isn't having some sort of reaction, your mind is swirling with all the wonderful things you recall from childhood that they now can't have. It's exhausting.

From discussions online and in support groups it's clear that, while labelling has improved dramatically in recent years, many people – manufacturers too – remain hopelessly confused by what the various statements mean. So, let's start with the law.

Food labelling – the law

Sometimes the world of food labelling seems to grind slowly, at other times there's a flurry of activity and we get a whole new set of rules and regulations. Things have been overhauled quite dramatically since we were first diagnosed.

In 2014, the Regulation (EU) No 1169/2011[1] directive came into effect, updating the requirement to list certain common allergens on all food labels and in all food settings. These are the fabled 'Top 14' as follows:

Eggs

Milk

Peanuts

Tree nuts (almonds, hazelnuts, walnuts, Brazil nuts, cashews, pecans, pistachios and macadamia nuts)

Sesame

Fish

Soya beans

Cereals containing gluten (wheat – such as spelt – rye, barley and oats)

Crustaceans (such as prawns, crabs and lobsters)

Molluscs (such as mussels and oysters)

Mustard

---

1 Regulation (EU) No 1169/2011 of the European Parliament and of the Council of 25 October 2011 on the provision of food information to consumers: <https://www.legislation.gov.uk/eur/2011/1169/contents>

Celery
Lupin
Sulphur dioxide and sulphites.

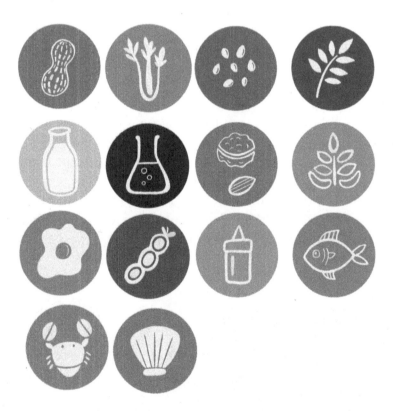

Adapted from Kath Grimshaw's book *The Cookie* published by Little Green Elephant Books <littlegreenelephantbooks.co.uk>.

There is some ongoing debate about whether other, increasingly common, allergens ought to be added to the list – kiwi, for example – but at the moment the Top 14 remains as it is.

Obviously, allergens are not isolated to these 'Top 14' and many people, and in particular children, are allergic to legumes such as chickpeas, peas or lentils. Others may be allergic to coconut or pine nut (not defined as 'tree nuts'), tomatoes and so on. It's one of the reasons I hate the term 'allergen free' that's sometimes misleadingly used on 'free from' foods as, frankly, there is no such thing.

The law states that, when present in the ingredients of a food product or dish, these 14 allergens must be emphasized on labelling – this may be in bold, underlined, italicized or in a different colour font. They also need to be large enough to be legible, easy to see, difficult to remove and not in any way hidden, obscured or detracted from.

When eating out or ordering food, the caterer is legally obliged to tell you if any of these 14 allergens are present in their dishes.

Exemptions to the Top 14

There are some derivatives of the Top 14 allergens that are so refined they are not perceived as posing a risk to people with allergies. These are exempt from having to be highlighted in the ingredients list. They include 'wheat-based glucose syrups' such as dextrose, 'wheat-based maltodextrins', fish gelatine used as a carrier in products including vitamins, 'fully refined soybean oil', and lactitol, which is derived from milk sugar.

Soya lecithin **does** have to be declared as, while many people with soya allergy can tolerate it, it is not suitable for all.

Does Brexit mean we lose these regulations?

Despite Brexit, the Food Standards Agency has confirmed that all EU laws on food labelling are being retained and written into UK legislation.

Pre-packed food

The 14 allergens must be emphasized within the ingredients list of pre-packed food or drink (that's the food you buy from shops and supermarkets in sealed packs, made in factories or facilities off-site). This can be done, for example, by using bold, italic or coloured type, to make the allergen ingredients easier to spot.

The 'contains' box

Before the 2014 EU regulations came in, manufacturers were allowed to include an allergen statement on their packaging that came to be known as the 'contains box'. It would be a box or highlighted section that read 'Contains nuts and milk', for example. This is no longer permitted – all allergens deliberately present **have** to be emphasized within the ingredients list, by law. The idea behind this is that all the allergen information will appear in one place only, to avoid confusion. A manufacturer can include a signposting statement instead, that could read something like: 'For allergens, please see ingredients in bold'.

Non-prepacked (loose) food

Food businesses such as bakeries, butchers or delicatessens must provide you with allergen information for any loose item you buy that contains any of the 14 allergens. This can be communicated in writing or verbally at point of sale.

Pre-packed for direct sale (PPDS)

From October 2021, food that is pre-packed for direct sale (PPDS) must have a label that displays a full ingredients list with the top 14 allergens emphasized within that list, if present.

The new PPDS food rules – also known as 'Natasha's Law' – are, in great part, a consequence of the powerful campaigning by the family of teenager Natasha Ednan-Laperouse, who tragically died in 2016 after unwittingly consuming sesame in a Pret A Manger baguette.

What is pre-packed for direct sale food?

This moniker basically means anywhere that **packages items on the premises ready for sale. They are packaged before the consumer chooses or buys them.**

This includes:

- sandwiches packed on-site and taken by the consumer from a chiller cabinet;
- salads displayed in deli boxes behind a counter and bought ready-to-go;
- takeaway items cooked and displayed in packaging on-site before purchase (e.g. pizza slices in a box or pre-wrapped burgers);
- supermarket foods such as weighed and packaged cheeses or meats; rotisserie chicken in a bag; or multi-packs of cakes or sausages packed on the premises.

It *doesn't* include foods that are prepared freshly to order and then wrapped or packaged to be taken away; or foods that are prepared in advance of a rush, displayed on the counter but not wrapped until they are bought by the consumer (e.g. a pile of filled bagels in a café). Yes, it's confusing.

The idea is that this will provide customers with more information, to make safe food choices. However, it should not replace or prevent consumers from having conversations with the food business about their allergy requirement.

Despite these new labelling rules, because these products will often be prepared and packaged freshly on-site it is incredibly important to ask staff about their allergen processes. Is there any risk of cross contamination, for example? These products will always be higher risk than pre-packed foods because of the way in which they are prepared, so it's important not to be complacent or to take the packaging at face value.

Distance selling or online orders

The 'PPDS' rules don't apply to businesses selling food online or by phone ('distance selling'). But they must give allergen information to consumers before they buy the product and again when the food is delivered.

While this information can be given in writing (e.g. on a website, a sticker, a menu or in a catalogue) it may also be provided orally, for example by phone, as long as the provider clearly flags up how the consumer is to access the information.

'May contain' labelling

Possibly the biggest minefield for allergy consumers is the issue of 'may contain' labelling. You may also hear this referred to as PAL ('precautionary allergen labelling'). These are the statements you will have seen on packs and in posters in restaurants or on menus stating something like, 'May contain traces of sesame' or 'Made in factory where milk is present'.

The idea is that it alerts customers to the fact that there may be small amounts of an allergen in the product. Contamination may happen unintentionally, or because there is a risk from shared production lines, or the supplier of an ingredient may declare there to be a risk from other foods it processes.

The problem with precautionary labelling is that it is **not currently covered by law**. Food Standards Agency guidance states that there must be a 'significant and demonstrable risk' of cross contamination – so the spirit of the guidance would warn against so-called 'blanket' labelling, a.k.a. back-covering, or legal disclaimers, where no genuine risk exists.

Food safety legislation (Regulation (EC) 852/2004) on hygiene also notes that precautionary labelling 'cannot be used as an excuse for a lack of good manufacturing practice, poor hygiene and sufficient control measures'.

What do the different statements mean?

There is a huge amount of misunderstanding out there about these labels. The first thing to know is that there is NO standardization when it comes to wording, and no hierarchy of risk.

What do I mean by that? Well, many people assume that a 'may contain milk' statement is automatically more of a risk than a 'made in a facility where milk is handled' statement. But there is no way of knowing whether this is the case or not.

Here are just some of the infinite variety of ways potential allergy cross contamination may be listed:

- May contain nuts
- May contain traces of nuts
- Made in a facility where nuts are processed
- Made in a factory where nuts are present
- Not suitable for nut allergy sufferers
- Packed in a facility which handles nuts
- Not suitable for customers with an allergy to nuts due to manufacturing methods
- Made in a premises that handles nuts
- Nuts are present in the manufacturing environment
- Produced on a line handling nuts
- Manufactured on equipment that processes nuts
- Made in a busy working kitchen so may contain traces of nuts and other allergens
- Our packing house handles nuts

Or, my personal favourite ...
- Due to the way our products are prepared, we can't guarantee the absence of nuts, eggs, sesame, milk, celery, lupin, eggs, fish, shellfish, wheat ...

The fact is, there are no rules on how a cross contamination risk has to be declared. These warnings may mean different levels of risk, or they may not. Without ringing a manufacturer and asking them to talk through their processes (which you can do) you can't make an accurate risk assessment based on what the labels actually say.

It's also important to note that once a manufacturer has placed any sort of warning label on their product, they have legally declared that risk. So it's perfectly possible that they may become complacent about allergen management processes, or that risk may vary during the course of a typical production period (milk may be processed on the same lines on some days, and others not).

Neither is it a good rule of thumb to assume that just because you have eaten a 'may contain' product safely many times before, it will always be so. The point about contamination is that it is not homogeneous, or equally distributed – in other words, 99 bites out of 100 you won't encounter anything. But, once out of 100 bites, you might.

A 2014 survey of allergen labelling and allergen content by the UK-based lab RSSL sampled various products for trace contamination.[2] It found 33 out of 542 products had detectable amounts of gluten, and 39 out of 474 had detectable amounts of milk. The highest risk products were found to be confectionery, with milk found at detectable levels in dark chocolate. The moral of that story is that if you are avoiding traces, any or all of the statements above are ones to watch.

Should I avoid 'traces'?

This book is not going to tell you 'you must avoid all traces' because every individual needs to make their own risk assessment, based on advice from their doctor.

I remember when we were first diagnosed, I asked our allergist whether we should be avoiding 'may contain' items. His answer wasn't black and white – and the truth is, there is no clear-cut answer. He said 50 per cent of his patients avoided

---

2 'Survey of allergen advisory labelling and allergen content of UK retail pre-packed processed foods', B. Hirst, RSSL, 2014. See: <https://www.food.gov.uk/sites/default/files/media/document/survey-allergen-labelling-prepacked.pdf>

them, and 50 per cent didn't. Which was true, and probably still holds true for the allergy community today.

There are very many people who believe they have reacted to traces. There are equally many allergists who say reactions to traces are 'as rare as hen's teeth' – or that the risk is minimal when you weigh up the burden of avoiding all 'may contains'.

How can you make that judgment, I hear you cry? It's probably been the single most confusing question of our allergy journey. Five people walk into a bar – an allergist, a food scientist, a dietitian, an allergic person and a food manufacturer – and you'll get a different answer from each. It's hugely stressful.

Even different medics take different views. One survey of doctors – including GPs and allergy specialists – found 32 per cent recommended complete avoidance of 'may contain nuts', 40 per cent advised there was no need to avoid foods with the warning, and the rest said avoid only under specific conditions.[3] As the study concluded: 'There are significant differences in the degree of avoidance recommended by medical professionals. The advice provided often contradicts the available literature on risks of allergic reaction with consumption of pre-packed foods. This can result in conflicting advice to patients and their families, and impact adversely upon their quality of life.' No shit, Sherlock, as they say.

Unfortunately, it only gets harder to assess risk when – as mentioned – manufacturers have no standardized way of declaring it. One manufacturer's 'may contain' does not equate to another's 'not suitable for'. One may be covering their back with a legal disclaimer when, in reality, there is no genuine risk, another will have commissioned an accredited lab to test

---

3 ''May contain traces' – what do doctors advise parents of food allergic children?', Turner et al, 2013. See (p.1466): <https://onlinelibrary.wiley.com/doi/epdf/10.1111/cea.12197>

for traces and imposed a precautionary label because there is a genuine concern about contamination.

As allergy parents we find ourselves well-versed in the intricacies of food production. Somehow I have acquired the knowledge that sesame is electrostatic and can go pinging around factories sticking to things. Some allergens are more 'sticky' or troublesome – such as chocolate, where milk contamination is a big issue, and where you can't rinse out the equipment with water because chocolate and water don't mix. Then again, you may be pretty safe to assume that a 'may contain nuts' statement on a bottle of orange squash is minimal risk.

Another study, by Brough et al[4] noted that some foods are higher risk for peanut contamination than others – with snack foods or speciality breads, for instance, being potentially more risky. But the study also posited that some consumption of 'may contains' may improve quality of life for a number of peanut allergic individuals – and that many already ignore precautionary statements on pre-packed foods without consequence. However, it added that it would be sensible to exercise caution 'when eating unfamiliar foods in an unfamiliar environment' or where medical support may be delayed or far away. The allergic individual should also be 'clinically well'.

Personally, our own approach is complicated. Mostly, I'd say we avoid traces. With sesame, 'may contain' is often on breads and baked goods and it seems to me that the risk of cross contamination in this context is pretty high. We never eat fresh baked products unless I've made them myself, or they are pre-packaged and from a manufacturer we trust. On the other hand, since outgrowing tree nut allergies we do try to keep those nuts in his diet, and so are often forced to consume tree

---

4 'Dietary management of peanut and tree nut allergy: what exactly should patients avoid?', Brough et al, *Clinical & Experimental Allergy*, 2014. See: <https://onlinelibrary.wiley.com/doi/pdf/10.1111/cea.12466>

nuts that are labelled with 'may contain traces of sesame and peanut'.

Where possible, we buy nuts in their shells but, frankly, shelling almonds nearly finished me off. As did the time we had a pine nut challenge at the hospital and I spent the night before shaving – yes, literally shaving – each individual pine nut to remove potential traces. There is a risk/benefit ratio here.

So, we have taken the decision to have tree nuts in the safety of our own home; never when travelling and never when out. Possibly we are more cautious than others, and over time we may relax our restrictions still further. But it works for us, so far. Each time, it's a fine balance of judgment, but the best way to approach it is armed with as much information as possible. Talk it through with your doctor and ask them to explain the reasoning behind their advice. Then you will be better placed to make your decision.

What to ask a manufacturer

Over time you will come to know and trust certain brands and retailers. Generally speaking, the supermarket own brands label very well. If a major UK supermarket has no 'may contain' on an own brand product I'm confident that it is safe to eat. I don't phone to check each item every time.

That's not to say I don't hate the precautionary labelling they stick on everything: you'll find you rely on one supermarket for a couple of years and then suddenly something or someone changes and they are slapping 'may contains' on previously safe products. It's infuriating, and it means you have to go to multiple shops to find what you need. (Top tip? Try not to get too attached to a single product. It's devastating when it disappears off your safe list and we've had this happen so many times now.)

Studies have shown that ordinary daily activities, such as grocery shopping, can dramatically impact upon quality of life for families with allergies – the need to visit several shops, check every label, track down 'safe' alternatives and so on. Shopping for a nut-allergic person is said to take almost 40 per cent longer and cost an average of 11 per cent more.[5]

Certain brands are very clear in their labelling and issue regular 'allergy safe lists'. Mondelez, which covers the likes of Cadbury and Oreo, are good – even better, the gold standard, they differentiate between 'nuts' (tree nuts) and 'peanuts', which is invaluable information for those who can eat one but not the other.

There are also certain 'free from' brands whose labelling is genuinely allergy friendly. Unfortunately, these smaller, independent brands come and go as supermarkets give them retail boosts then drop them at a whim. Some good places to look for safe brands include:

Nut Free Living

This online marketplace sells a growing range of nut free snacks and confectionery. It was set up by Angela Waters, whose daughter has nut allergies. She also runs a hugely helpful Facebook forum identifying nut-free products across UK retail. Visit <nutfreeliving.co.uk>.

The Free From Food Awards

These annual awards have been running for some years now, and I'm honoured to say I've been a judge since our son was small. It covers a wide range of 'free from' needs, including vegan and coeliac, but a browse of the website for winners and runners-up often throws up some great new allergy-friendly finds. Visit <freefromfoodawards. co.uk>.

Online stores

Try The Vegan Kind <thevegankindsupermarket.com> and Goodness Direct <goodnessdirect.co.uk> for some not-always-widely-available

---

5 'Dietary management of peanut and tree nut allergy: what exactly should patients avoid?', Brough et al, *Clinical & Experimental Allergy*, 2014. See: <https://onlinelibrary.wiley.com/doi/pdf/10.1111/cea.12466>

allergy-friendly brands. (Remember: vegan doesn't mean allergy friendly, so check the labels.)

'Free from' brands

These come and go, and I will no doubt have missed a great many, but for allergy-friendly treats there are a few that we often enjoy. Lazy Day Foods <lazydayfoods.com> make a range of 'free from' cakes and treats; Ananda <anandafoods.co.uk> makes egg, milk, nut and some gluten-free chocolate marshmallow snacks and cookies; the Just Love Food Co <justlovefoodcompany.com> has a range of variously egg, milk, gluten and nut free cakes – some of which are available in the supermarkets. For chocolate, try Nomo <nomochoc. com>, Berkleys Nut Free Chocolates <berkleysnutfreechocolates. co.uk>, Cocoa Libre <cocoalibre.co.uk>, Plamil <plamilfoods.co.uk> and D&D Chocolates <danddchocolates.com>.

FoodMaestro

This is a really handy app launched with the backing of allergy doctors and dietitians. You can plug in the foods you need to avoid and it has a database of products that meet your needs, from some of the leading UK supermarkets. It's not a replacement for label-checking but it does help to pull out some safe options you may not otherwise be aware of. See <foodmaestro.me>.

Nut (and some-nut) free butters

There are two nut-free spreads that many allergy families often use to replace conventional nut butters. Wowbutter <wowbutter.com> is a peanut and tree nut-free soya-based spread that you can find online and in many supermarkets. And the US-branded Sunbutter <sunbutter.com> is also free from many of the top allergens – it's made of sunflower seeds. Unfortunately, this isn't widely available in the UK but you can find it on a few online sites.

Barney Butter <barneybutter.com> is an almond butter that's peanut free and also free from other common tree nuts – helpful if you are trying to keep almonds in an otherwise allergic child's diet. And on a slight side note, in the UK Zeina Foods <zeinafoods.com> sells tree nuts in bags that are peanut, sesame and dairy free. (Given brands can change, do make sure to check the websites for all these products and the labels, too.)

Pick up the phone

Of course, there will always be a manufacturer you haven't yet tried and the only way to find out if they're safe for your child is to call them. Some will be great and quick in their responses; others either won't respond or will fudge their answers. You'll begin by spending hours on the phone and on email trying to establish whether an ice cream is safe. By the time you get a reply it'll be November and too cold for an ice cream anyway.

What should you be asking?

- Is there any risk of cross contamination from [state your allergen]?
- What is this risk? (Trust me – it's worth clarifying. A cake decoration company I am loyal to, to this day, for the honesty of their response once admitted that the 'may contain nut' label on their product was due to the 'peanut butter in the rat poison placed around the factory'. I kid you not. I judged the risk to be small.)
- What processes do you use to judge that risk? Are you assessed by an accredited lab?
- Will you use 'may contain' labelling if that risk changes?

An accredited lab would be one that meets certain rigorous standards – and they would be accredited in the UK by UKAS, the United Kingdom Accreditation Service, and/or internationally under ISO (International Organisation for Standardization) 17025.

You should also clarify that you are asking this question on behalf of someone with a serious food allergy, to be sure they don't minimize risk in their response. Unfortunately, you may also find they exaggerate risk out of fear – particularly if they are a small brand – but I guess it's better to be safe than sorry.

The Food Standards Agency, Anaphylaxis Campaign and Allergy UK all run a free food allergy alert service – if you subscribe to their emails they send out alerts when a product has had to be recalled or withdrawn due to allergen labelling or contamination issues. You can sign up via their websites.

Vegan doesn't mean allergy safe

One of the biggest mistakes people make is to assume that 'vegan' products are also safe for those with, for example, milk, fish and egg allergies.

In fact, a 'vegan' label does not mean free from traces. As the Vegan Society states: 'The Vegan Society is not against foods labelled as vegan also carrying a 'may contain' warning about animal allergens … The Vegan Society does not claim that products registered with the Vegan trademark are suitable for people with allergies.'

The Food and Drink Federation also notes: 'There is a clear risk to allergic consumers who treat "vegan" claims and allergen absence claims (e.g. milk free) as equivalent, and this has potential serious health implications. It is therefore important that allergic consumers do not automatically assume that products labelled as "vegan" are suitable for them.'

The same applies when eating out – ordering a vegan item from a menu is not the same as asking for that item to be made safe for someone with an allergy.

Allergy free, 14 allergens free, free from and other claims

You may find a variety of claims on food products, ranging from 'allergen free' to 'free from', 'allergy safe' or '14 allergens free'. 'Allergen free' is a big gripe of mine, as it's not possible – and implies the only allergens are those in the 'Top 14'.

There is a strict definition when it comes to foods that actively make a 'free from' claim. If they state 'dairy free', for example, or 'nut free', this means that:

- Only 'free-from' materials have been used in the product recipe or in manufacture.
- The manufacturing environment has been strictly managed so as to eliminate risk of allergen cross contamination.
- There should be a 'robust sampling and testing programme' in place.

This doesn't mean that allergic consumers can only eat foods defined as 'free from', or 'x allergen free'. A product that doesn't contain your allergen, and where cross contamination has been judged unlikely or is properly managed, will also be safe to eat.

Thresholds

There is an awful lot of work going on into thresholds – that is, the specific quantity of an allergenic protein required to trigger an allergic reaction.

Currently only gluten and sulphites have thresholds defined in law. A food can be labelled as being 'gluten free' if it contains 20 parts per million or less of gluten. The Coeliac Society recognizes this as being a safe level for all people following a gluten-free diet. The same applies to sulphites at 10mg per kg.

In Australia, the food industry body The Allergen Bureau is spearheading something called VITAL (Voluntary Incidental Trace Allergen Labelling). An expert panel is developing threshold doses for the major allergens that can feed into the way manufacturers use 'may contain' labelling. Some manufacturers have already implemented the new thresholds, but these are not yet legislated for in the UK.

The global food standards body Codex Alimentarius is working with national partners, including the Food Standards

Agency, to harmonize allergen threshold levels so a new international standard can guide 'may contains' labelling.

One difficulty is the gap between what analytical studies find, and what the clinical outcome would be – for example, a genuinely trace amount of a certain allergen may be found in manufacture, but would it actually cause a reaction among the vast majority of allergic consumers?

Can we find a reliable and affordable way to test food, that can be used by all manufacturers – and by enforcement officers when needed? Would these tests work on all types of food? All these questions are being interrogated now.

9

Preparing food at home

It becomes second nature soon enough, but rethinking the way you shop, prep, store and cook takes a while to bed in. Hopefully this chapter will help to make the new regime a little easier.

Should I remove all allergens from the house?

This is another tricky and personal one. It's clearly much easier to remove sesame from the house than it is wheat, or milk. For many families juggling different dietary needs, or non-allergic siblings, keeping key food groups on the go for everyone else may be important.

Many families designate a cupboard or a shelf in the fridge either for 'safe' or 'non-safe' products. As I said earlier, we often have a jar of peanut butter way up out of reach above the ironing board cupboard for our littlest to have, now and again. My mother wraps all things eggy – mayonnaise, tartare sauce – in cling film in the fridge when we visit. My sister has a 'safe drawer' for when we go round – flour, snacks, chocolates, jams, all unsullied by potential allergens.

A family will make different judgments based on the allergen in question. The key thing is making sure to prevent mix-ups or spillages, in whichever way you see fit. Perhaps you might start cautiously and introduce allergens to the home as your child gets older, and everyone gets more of a handle on what can and can't be eaten.

Simplicity and clarity are key – a separate shelf or drawer, a colour-coding system, or just labelling everything that's either safe, or unsafe. Plus either separating utensils or making sure surfaces, equipment and hands are thoroughly washed when prepping food and before and after eating. Here's how other allergy families tackle it:

'My son has his own 'dairy free' shelf in the fridge, his own drawer in the freezer and his own shelves and labelled snack boxes in the cupboard. We all use dairy-free spread to avoid mix-ups and I cook gluten-free pasta for everyone for simplicity. We have separate utensils and pans for cooking and use different coloured plates and cutlery. My son's are all blue.'

'Eldest is allergic to milk and egg. I have both in the house, in a second small fridge and usually only eaten at breakfast. I'm strict with his siblings – they can only eat at the table and wash hands afterwards. All family meals or other foods bought are allergy safe, and if not we label them clearly with a Sharpie.'

'Two out of four of us is coeliac. We have one cupboard with glutenous bread and other bits, plus separate butters and toasters. The rest of the kitchen is gluten free. We make sure to wash utensils properly. You get used to it – practise makes perfect!'

'For twins – one with allergies, one without – we use different coloured bottles, cups, lunchboxes, or label them to ensure one can still have dairy. We have a shelf in the fridge and cupboard with 'safe' alternatives and snacks for the allergic child.'

'We do have some items that are 'may contains' and one or two other things with her allergens in, but we ask that our daughter always checks everything and the 'worst' allergens we don't consume at home. Peanut butter, definitely not – too easy to spread on surfaces for cross contamination.'

'My son has his own shelf in the fridge so cheese and so on is kept away. He also checks his food – every label, every time.'

'We are a nut-free household but we do have his other allergens, eggs, dairy, fish and legumes, in the house. We prepare his food separately and first.'

'We all eat the same foods at home, for inclusion and safety. Younger sibling gets to eat allergic treats away from home if he wants and decontaminates afterwards!'

How to minimise cross contamination when catering – your step-by-step guide

The battle to convince more people to cater for food allergies is double-edged. On the one hand, you want to show how simple it can be – some common sense, a clean kitchen and utensils, and being scrupulous about ingredients does the trick. On the other hand, it's vital to stress how dangerous it can be if those simple processes aren't undertaken properly.

I understand why many run scared. Legally, it's virtually impossible for anyone to describe their premises as 100 per cent guaranteed 'nut free'. But it *is* possible to cater safely for both allergic and non-allergic guests.

Here are some steps to follow when catering for food allergies. I wrote a blog post on this years ago when my son was very small. The next time we visited my mother-in-law, she had printed it out and stuck it to her kitchen pinboard. Lovely!

1 **Use only scrupulously clean utensils.** I prefer not to use wooden spoons or boards as they soak up oils. Everything else I wash well with washing up liquid and water (which is enough to get rid of allergenic proteins) or on a hot dishwasher setting.
2 **Use clean dishcloths and tea towels.**
3 **Don't use any cooking gear that has a patina of food still on it** (e.g. cast iron pans, ancient baking trays, oven

shelves). Make sure you wash thoroughly any extra pieces of equipment you may be using (food processors, scales, grill pans etc.).

4   **Wash down all surfaces with soap and hot water.** Dry with a clean cloth.

5   If in doubt, **line a baking tray or oven shelf with baking paper or foil,** or use a disposable foil baking tray.

6   When preparing the dish, **keep all other allergens away** – e.g. don't try to prepare a gluten-free dish at the same time as you prepare a floury cake.

7   **Store allergy friendly ingredients in a separate cupboard.** Gluten-free flour should not be stored next to gluten-containing flour, for instance.

8   **Use butter, cheese, jam, yoghurt, sugar, flour etc. that has not been contaminated with any other knife/spoon.** This counts for every item, from salt to herbs, spices and condiments. **If you can, buy fresh and use a new one.** Store it in a closed container away from other items, clearly labelled. Ensure a clean knife or spoon is used every time.

9   **Never re-use cooking oil.**

10 **Check the label** on every item of food you use – ensure there are no allergens listed and no 'traces' warnings. **If in doubt, ask the person you are catering for** whether they are happy for you to use that product, **or ring the manufacturer** to check there is no cross-contamination.

11 Finally – **wash your hands thoroughly and keep washing them throughout.** Use a soap that doesn't have the avoided allergen as an ingredient. **Wear a clean apron** and ensure you don't have any remnants of food on your clothes. Don't snack on anything while preparing the food, and **if you need to taste anything use a clean spoon** and put it straight in the dishwasher/sink after tasting.

If that sounds arduous, have another read and consider which steps you would undertake when cooking for others anyway. Presumably (hopefully) you would use clean utensils, wipe down the kitchen and wash your hands first. Catering for food allergies means being more methodical and scrupulous than you would ordinarily be, but if you keep this check list to hand and stick to it, you really can't go far wrong.

Last note: when the food is done, if it's not being served up immediately (on a clean plate!) then store it in a closed container, away from all other foods and clearly labelled. When serving, use a clean knife/spoon.

10

Eating out

The big leap

When you are still reeling from diagnosis, the very notion of ever letting anyone prepare food for your child again is ... difficult. I'll preface this section by saying we ate nowhere outside our home until maybe two or three years into our allergy journey.

That was the wonderful allergy-friendly, kid-centred Higher Lank Farm down in Cornwall, where we knew other friends with allergies had visited safely and where we preceded our visit with dozens of calls and emails back and forth. So my number one piece of advice is ...

- **Don't feel pressurized into eating out.** This one's a biggie. It took me some time, because I needed to get to a stage where I was feeling more confident about managing my son's allergies, and had a grip on exactly which foods he was allergic to.

Other allergy parents can sometimes be a bit (well-meaningly) pushy about eating out – they do it, and are understandably keen to encourage others, but it has to be a step taken when you feel the time is right.

I do think it's important to get there at some point: I wanted us as a family to be able to go out to eat, for my son to enjoy great food (I'm a decent cook but there's a limit), have a future with a full social life and, vitally, to hear us asking all the questions he will need to ask, and taking all the precautions he will need to take, as he gets older. I started tentatively at one or two places on the recommendations of a fellow allergy parent, whose opinion I trusted, and built my confidence from there.

Finding safe spots isn't always easy, but you will build up a small roster of tried and trusted favourites. There are some chains that have excellent systems and procedures, and smaller independents that just have very lovely, thorough management and chefs. You will find them. In your own time.

The Rules

Before you do eat out, though, there are The Rules. They are the steps we take, and the key things we consider. Here goes:

- **Check the menu online** and get a sense of what the restaurant serves. Very often you'll find information on their allergen processes here, too.
- **I always ring and email in advance** to check the manager and chef are aware, and in some cases we pre-order our meal. It starts as a sussing-out call – do they sound as if they know what they're doing? If not, forget it. If they do, I'll go into greater detail, stress that we need the food to be prepped free from cross contamination, and find out what dishes are likely to be safe for my son to eat.
- **I go through every ingredient** – flour, oil, gravy stock, even cheese – to ensure none is a 'may contain' product and we won't unwittingly be fed, for instance, Grana Padano (contains egg) instead of Parmesan.
- **Ask if the person you have spoken to will be present** and, if not, ask for the details of someone who will be and request that they are also fully versed in everything you've discussed.
- **Follow up with an email to confirm** everything you have agreed and ordered, and to reiterate again your child's allergies and the need to avoid cross contamination.

- Upon arrival I always repeat the 'can you prep my son's meal without cross contamination?' spiel and make sure whoever is serving us is fully briefed.
- I prefer it if the manager on duty serves us directly and if we can at some point – in advance or on arrival – have a conversation with the chef, too.
- If you find a safe chain, don't assume every branch is equally sussed – you'll have to go through the same rigmarole in every branch, as standards can vary enormously.
- Similarly, if you find a safe place to eat, remind them of your needs each time you visit. Staff change, recipes change: you can never be complacent.
- Ask that the waiting staff note down your allergies when you order – it's an extra check and balance.
- Try to go for off-peak times – a midday lunch, for example, or a 5pm tea. Easy when the kids are small and it fits their routine, but it's probably a good idea to aim for the quieter periods where possible: the start of a lunch or evening service is a good slot.
- Factor in a longer wait as allergy-friendly food will often have to be prepped from scratch. I take sticker books. That may not work when he's 15.
- Try to help a restaurant by spelling out what you can have, not just what you can't. If meat and two veg is generally a safe option, or a simple tomato pasta dish, let them know so they can think up something that works for their kitchen. Make it easier for them – it's not their job to guess what we need.
- Draw your own parameters. For me, the existence of nuts or eggs on a restaurant menu does not signify an automatic no-no. But I will always ask how a restaurant manages cross contamination, and specifically in relation to dishes that give cause for concern. But don't be swayed by others' opinions – stay within

your personal comfort zone. Ask all the right questions and expect all the right answers, otherwise ...

- ... my absolute rule of thumb is: **any doubts? Don't do it.**

Other than all of that, bear in mind: puddings may more often than not be fruit salad (it's time to celebrate when a chef goes to the trouble of whipping up a whole safe pudding). Bread and breadsticks are usually a no-no (risk of cross contamination with nuts and sesame) so I bring some if I think they might be asked for. And if the rest of us might want to order dessert, I bring a safe cake or chocolate treat for my son to have, too.

If that bumper list doesn't make it clear, going out for a meal with allergies is far from spontaneous. And if, like me, you favour skulking anonymously into a restaurant to hunker down without fuss, get used to never being able to do this again.

Expert advocate, researcher and trainer in allergy risks Dr Hazel Gowland notes: 'There are no shortcuts – you have to do the journey, you have to do the risk assessment and negotiate that.'

But it's worth it.

What the law says – what information a restaurant has to give you

So what's the lowdown on what you can rightly expect when eating out? You can find all the guidance via the Food Standards Agency at <food.gov.uk>, but here's a summary so you can make the leap fully armed:

First things first – when you eat out, or order a takeaway, the restaurant or café **must provide you with allergen information.** This could be on their menu, on a chalkboard, in an information pack, or via a written notice explaining how you can obtain the information ('please ask a member of staff about allergens in our food'). This notice must be 'placed in a clearly visible position'.

If allergen information is provided as part of a conversation with a customer (the 'please speak to a member of staff' way of doing things), it would be good practice – although not a legal requirement – to back that up with written info, to ensure it's 'accurate and consistent'.

Restaurants have to tell you which, if any, of the 'Top 14' allergens are present in the food (see Chapter 8). They do not have to give you information about 'may contains' – but you will find some well-known chains offer this information. Nando's, for example, is well-known for producing a regularly-updated allergen booklet that lists all allergens and risks of contamination for each item on the menu.

Food businesses are not, however, obliged to offer you an alternative meal to meet your requirements.

A quick reminder to:

- Call ahead where possible to ask what their allergy policy is.
- Be clear about your allergy when making your order – give examples of the foods that cause your child a reaction.
- Ask them how they manage the risk of cross contamination.
- If you don't feel the member of staff you are speaking to understands your needs, ask to speak to the manager.
- Leave if you don't feel comfortable or that they are not taking your needs seriously.

Questions to ask

- Do you offer meals that are suitable for my child?
- If not, are you able to make a safe dish?
- How is the food handled in the kitchen – is there a chance of allergen cross contamination from cooking equipment or ingredients?

- Has there been a last-minute recipe change or ingredient substitution?
- Remind them to be careful of cross contamination or added allergens from glazes, toppings, sauces and cooking oils.

Buffets

Allergen information must be provided separately for each dish on a buffet – not just for the buffet as a whole. Again, this could be by labelling the allergens in each dish or by displaying a clearly visible and legible sign directing customers to ask staff for allergen information.

Having said this, buffets are very risky for allergic consumers, given the high probability of cross contamination, and so I would tend to avoid them. Staff may bring out unused versions of safe dishes for your child rather than serve you from the main area. It's always a delight when we encounter a breakfast buffet with safe cereal in a closed mini packet – a variety pack of Cornflakes or a twin pack of Weetabix can make our day. Pleasures come simple when you've got allergies to deal with.

Watch out for complicated dishes

Complex dishes can contain hidden allergens, so this requires a conversation about every element of the meal. Often it may be preferable to opt for a simple dish with few sauces or 'extras' – although you should always check ingredients for everything from gravy to seasoning.

Takeaways

Ordering a takeaway is considered 'distance selling' (see Chapter 8). Allergen info must be made available to the consumer at the point of selection – so before you order it – and again when it is delivered. This info can be given in writing (for example, online, in a booklet or on a menu) or orally, by phone. But you should be clearly signposted to where you can find it through notices on the website, app, menu and in-store. The same allergen info must be provided again when the food is delivered, in writing (for example, using allergen stickers or via an enclosed menu with allergens listed for each item) or, again, by phone.

If you are ordering for more than one person, ask the restaurant to clearly label each meal and container so you know which order is suitable for those with an allergy. This should also indicate that additional controls have been applied to prevent allergen cross contamination on that product or dish.

It can often be safer to order and collect takeaways in person rather than to rely on delivery drivers, or 'middle man' companies and apps such as Just Eat or Deliveroo. Some brands have made the decision not to cater for allergies on orders placed through delivery, because of the inherent risks.

Many allergy families build up a personal relationship with a tried and trusted local, and ring ahead to place their order and have a full discussion with the manager. When having that conversation, make sure you cover both the food allergens you need to avoid, and additional steps needed to prevent allergen contamination.

How do I deal with being asked to sign a waiver?

Ugh. There's been a spate of reports in recent years of restaurants and pubs asking allergic consumers to sign waivers before eating. Don't do it.

Food Standards Agency advice is: 'Food businesses cannot avoid or limit their legal responsibility to provide safe food and accurate allergen info by asking customers to sign waivers. If you are asked to sign a waiver because you have a food allergy, we recommend that you do not do so.'

What about 'we cannot guarantee' disclaimers everywhere?

It's hugely infuriating and sometimes upsetting to walk into a restaurant or speak to a manager and be met with a big old 'we cannot guarantee any of our dishes are allergen free' – whether that's a massive red sign or a pre-rehearsed verbal spiel.

Unfortunately, you'll find an awful lot of this and to an extent it's understandable. There *are* no cast iron guarantees, and everything is a balance of risk and careful management. It comes down to the conversation you have with the person in charge on the day. If they can't talk you through their processes for managing contamination, and just keep repeating the same disclaimers, my instinct would be to leave. If they acknowledge there is never a 100 per cent guarantee but can explain all the steps they will take to keep your food from being contaminated, then that's much better.

Personally, I love the sort of statement you find in allergy-friendly chains such as Wagamama, whose online allergen guide states: 'We want everyone to be able to enjoy Wagamama … if you don't find the information you need or are at all unsure just ask a member of our team … We are able to modify some recipes to remove or replace certain ingredients and try to be as flexible as possible.' They still have the line: 'Whilst we try our best to ensure your food is suitable for you, our dishes are prepared in areas in which allergenic ingredients are present'. It's the truth, but if their systems are good, it's a manageable risk.

As is the case every time you eat out, it's all about clear communication, on both sides.

Look out for hidden allergens

There are certain cuisines and dishes that may pose a particularly high risk for those with allergies. For example:

- Asian food – e.g. Indian, Chinese, Vietnamese – very often contains nuts and nut oils, or sesame.
- Shared frying oil can be a risk, such as in fish and chip shops – ask if your order will be prepared in a fryer with clean oil, and separately from your allergens (remember egg in batter, nut or sesame oils, gluten in crumb coatings and so on).
- Woks and frying pans may pose a risk if the business isn't using a fresh pan for your order.
- Sauces may contain hidden allergens such as wheat flour, or butter, or may be thickened with peanut or almond flour.
- Breads and crackers may contain nuts or seeds.
- Don't assume a dish you've eaten before is safe – recipes vary depending on the venue, the chef and ingredients available on the day.

B.Y.O.

Granted, this one is easier with little kids but sometimes you may be in a situation where a restaurant can't cater, or you just don't feel comfortable, but for whatever reason you still need or want to go. Perhaps you are meeting friends or family at short notice, or want to stop off spontaneously in a café or pub but don't think they can cater.

If we can, we phone in advance, explain the situation, and ask if they would mind if we brought an allergy-safe packed lunch for our son. Generally people are really kind and accommodating and will appreciate your nervousness or caution.

Or, if we are stopping somewhere impromptu – a café while on a long walk, or out shopping – we always explain our situation to the manager and ask if they would mind if we gave our son a sandwich or treat brought from home.

The only time we've ever met resistance has been a tiny English tearoom in the ruins of a castle – we bought copious pots of tea and slices of cake for ourselves and our daughter, and asked the owner if he would mind if we gave our son a safe jam tart from home. He refused. Sometimes you just encounter difficult people.

A chef's view

Dominic Teague, executive chef at London hotel One Aldwych, introduced a completely dairy- and gluten-free menu to his Indigo restaurant several years ago – without telling anyone.

'We were having a refit anyway and at that point allergies weren't necessarily being taken as seriously as they are now and I thought, "can people not go out for a nice meal? That's not on",' he recalls. 'Demand was growing but I didn't want to seem to be jumping on a bandwagon, so we just did it without any fanfare. We are a great restaurant, full stop, we just happen to be dairy and gluten free. And people didn't even notice – we'd tell them at the end and they'd say, "what, really?"'

The restaurant makes everything from scratch, from bread to dairy-free spread and ice creams. He says the difficulty for many kitchens is often that food – sauces, soups and purees, for example – is pre-prepared, so walking in off the street and asking for a meal to be served without certain allergens can be tricky, especially at busy times. 'Obviously things like meat and fish are prepared to order, but all the other bits and bobs around are normally ready, so it poses a challenge.'

The food industry is also a 'vast one', he adds, 'so at one end there's a chef like myself with 30 years' experience and a well-paid team in a great hotel, and at the other there's a café down the road. The question is how do we level it out across the whole industry?'

Teague is a big advocate for an audited allergen rating scheme that sits independently of the Food Standards Agency's food hygiene scores. He would also like standardized allergy training:

'Until you, the consumer, can go into a restaurant and ask, do you have Level 1* certification, how do you know?'

While many chains can handle big menus and have allergen control procedures put in place by 'armies' of people who audit and inspect, he says as a general rule it's good to think, 'less is more'. 'I'd look at a place with a massive menu and alarm bells would ring straight away, because there's so much more chance of error. Also, less is more when you're in a restaurant and it's really busy: I would be inclined to choose the simple dishes – you've got less going on the plate and less chance to go wrong.'

Organizing a meal in advance, if possible, takes the pressure off everyone, Teague adds: 'At our level we make it happen but it's always much easier if we have that conversation before someone comes in.'

Dealing with single allergies without advance notice is manageable, but the task becomes more complicated when there are multiple allergies to manage. He says: 'It's all relative. If it's Monday night and there are three tables, it's very different to a packed Saturday night.'

Here are some more of his top tips:

'Make contact beforehand if you have time and see what sort of response you get. If they seem to know what they are talking about and embrace the conversation that's a positive. If you get a wishy-washy answer, I wouldn't go there.'

'Go straight to the senior person and say, "I'd like to be served by a manager or assistant manager". That should really be happening anyway if they are taking allergy seriously.'

'Ask for some explanation of the system they have in place. If you're asking something like, "how do you handle nuts in your kitchen?", I'd be looking for an answer like, "we do have nuts but

they are stored separately in closed containers, and they are only used in one dessert". You want to know they know the detail.'

'Ask to see the allergen chart – wherever you are eating out, you can ask to see this, it's your right. And if they have one readily available that should show you whether they are taking allergies seriously or not.'

'Consider asking things like how long has the chef been here, have they done allergen training, or do they have any online certification? It's another layer to know. It's about trying to identify how serious they are.'

'Staff turnover may be high, a new chef may be in place – even if you've been somewhere before, have that same conversation every time.'

'It's always OK to check. If someone brings something over to your table it's OK to ask again – making sure this is the fish and chips with no egg, or whatever it may be. I know it must be an absolute pain for you but, from our side, we would always prefer that than a customer didn't say anything and a mistake was made.'

'If you're getting the sense that they don't want to do the checks then that's a signal to me that they don't deserve your money.'

'If language is an issue ask to speak to someone else, and it's always OK to ask to speak to the chef. We have to get to the point where it's normal from both sides and I think it will get to that.'

He adds: 'The vast majority of places do what we do because we enjoy it, it's our job and we want to do it properly. It's OK to keep checking, it's OK because we'd rather that and you have a good time. At the end of the day you're still paying good money – it's not like we're doing you a favour.' And if you're still feeling nervous? 'Do some research, look online, look at social media and see what's been said. It's a case of getting a feel for a place and making contact and building a relationship and a rapport. Have the confidence and remember that, if they take it seriously, they should be able to answer and bat your concerns away with no drama. If they aren't happy to answer, then that's a red flag.'

Take a chef card

The Food Standards Agency has downloadable 'chef card' that can help you when ordering in a restaurant. It has space for you to list your allergens and explains: 'Please let me know if my meal contains these ingredients. Just a small amount could make me very ill.' Find it here: <https://www.food.gov.uk/sites/default/files/media/document/allergy-chef-cards.pdf>.

How to report problems or make a complaint

If you come across a business that isn't meeting allergen regulations or fails to give you the information you need, the first step is to speak to the manager and see if they are willing and able to amend the mistakes. If this isn't possible, if they aren't amenable, or if you feel the issue merits investigation, you should contact the relevant Local Authority (LA) to report the problem. The Food Standards Agency (FSA) advises consumers to contact the council where the food business you are reporting is located. If you are unsure which Local Authority the business falls under, head to the FSA website (at <food.gov.uk>) where you can enter the name and address to find the contact details of the LA best suited to deal with your complaint.

Bear in mind that there is variability across the UK, and you may find you are instead asked to report the issue to the council where you live. Either way, you will need to speak to the Environmental Health department or Trading Standards, who have the power to investigate and enforce the law. You should find all the contact numbers and email addresses you need on the council website. Even if you give them a ring first, it's a good idea to report via email as this provides a written trail.

As a very general rule, Trading Standards deals with labelling problems and misdescribed food, while Environmental Health deals with food hygiene and food safety issues. If you hit any hurdles, try the Citizens Advice Bureau at <citizensadvice.org.uk> or call their helpline on 0808 223 1133.

Unfortunately, the system for reporting isn't always user friendly and can be a bit circuitous, and sometimes frustrating, but it is worth it. I have done this on one or two occasions – when a café seemed blissfully unaware that almonds were tree nuts, and labelled an almond milk-containing cake as being nut free (when I say unaware, I had a heated debate with the manager who swore blind almond milk didn't count); and again when I watched a member of staff at a café handle raw eggs and customers' change without washing his hands in between.

If your report is urgent – you have had a reaction or you think the business poses an immediate danger – you should obviously first and foremost deal with the reaction as your allergy care plan advises. If possible, keep a sample of the food as this may be the only way to later find out what caused the reaction. Let the restaurant know that your child is having or has had an allergic reaction and ask them to check what was in the food – they may need to contact suppliers.

If you suspect the food has been misdescribed, mislabelled or they haven't taken your allergy needs into account, you should:

- Prepare a report of the incident, including details of how you chose your meal, who you spoke to, what information you sought and were given.
- Think about timings and try to include these where possible.
- If you have a food sample, double wrap it in clean cling film and/or a plastic bag, label it and freeze it.

Make a formal written complaint to the business and report the issue directly to the Environmental Health or Trading Standards as described above. Depending on the response, you may also want to seek the advice of a patient organization, such as the Anaphylaxis Campaign, or even take legal advice. You should consider reporting any allergic reaction to your family doctor or allergy clinic. If it's a serious issue, putting others at risk, it may also be worth flagging directly with the Food Standards Agency too.

11

Party planning and events

One of my most vivid memories from when my son was tiny is of going to a first birthday party – possibly even our very first 'first birthday' party – and the parents wheeling out the most beautiful, bright, jolly yellow duck cake. While the other babies shovelled up the sponge and jam with fat, happy hands, our little one busied himself – quite contentedly, I have to say – with sticks of boiled courgette (I know, I know, but I hadn't anticipated the cake thing and it was all I had to hand ...).

I'd probably be lying if I said parties had got easier since then. But I have got a whole lot better at anticipating what might happen and providing for all eventualities. He's into double figures now, and we haven't had to send him to any more birthdays with boiled courgette.

Going to a party – checklist

There will be all sorts of parties, from baby birthdays to family weddings, school discos and beyond. The first and most important rules of thumb are:

- Always carry your medication. Consider this the golden rule for every single activity you ever do. If you leave your med pack at home, go back and get it. If you lose your med pack, get yourself an emergency replacement (see Chapter 2).
- Pack all the food you need for the occasion. Even if the event organizer has assured you that safe food will be provided, take enough safe snacks to get you through in an emergency.
- Take something to wipe down surfaces and clean hands.

What can I ask of the host?

Look, the truth is that what we all really want to do is reply to any party invitation with a five-page pamphlet outlining our child's allergies and laying out exactly which foods and activities we would please like removed from a five-mile surrounding radius, thank you. And here's a recipe for a four-tier nut, egg, gluten, dairy and soya-free cake, with allergy-friendly frosting. And, while you're at it, this is what we can and can't have in the party bags, OK? And, no, you can't put that in the piñata.

In reality, we have to be a bit more amenable if we are ever going to be invited to a party again.

Here's how to respond to a party invitation:

- Don't panic. This is a nice thing! Your child has been invited to a party (I know too well that stomach-sinking feeling, just when you should be feeling all peppy and pleased).
- Talk to the host and explain your child would love to go but he or she has food allergies, so you need to check a few things in advance (think: what food will be served? Any treats for prizes or party bags? Any other food-related activities?).
- Explain you are happy to bring your child's food and treats, you just need to be aware of any risks in advance.
- If it's an external venue, call them up and check on the menu. You may even find they can cater or substitute safe items on the menu for your child.

With toddlers, the situation is probably more critical, given they spend their time crawling on the floor, smooshing their fists into bowls of snacks, biting one another's noses and throwing bananas. It's an allergy alert zone. When our son was very small, we would ask friends with young children if they would mind very much not having his allergens within grabbing distance, or not making them available to the kids.

We never demanded that the food on-site would necessarily be completely safe for him to eat – it felt a bit much to be insisting on no traces, or instructing party hosts on how to prepare food in their own kitchens. Instead, we would ask – and still ask to this day – for a list of the food they were planning to provide and we would bring a pack matching the treats, as far as possible.

It's happy days when the party fare is old-school sandwiches, pizza, crisps and jelly. I can't tell you the preparation that went into the time we were told Brazilian cheese puffs and a unicorn cake were on the menu …

Template text

Sometimes emails, texts and conversations where you have to bring up your child's allergies and ask for accommodations can be so tricky. I know I've mithered over messages, finessing the wording, adding an extra 'sorry' and another 'thanks' so as not to come off all pushy.

You'll have your own way of communicating but, if you're stuck, this template text reply to a party invitation might be a handy springboard. It has the added bonus of letting you find out what food will be served ahead of time, so if there are any worries about allergens on the menu you can raise them early:

> *Hi x and thanks so much for the party invitation – x would love to come! I'm not sure if you know, but x has severe food allergies to x, y and z, so we'll be bringing his food along with him, if that's OK? Whenever you get a sec, would you mind letting me know what the menu is, just so I can try to match it? Thank you – x is very excited!*

Things to remember

Parties in soft play centres and other public places can be a headache on top of the usual. But it's important to know they are generally perfectly manageable.

Get used to the fact that you will be wiping hands and hovering while your child is still young as, with the best will in the world, someone will always be careering around with a peanut puff or squeezy yoghurt. This doesn't mean these parties are inherently dangerous. They're just a bit more work than we'd all envisaged pre-kids (no lounging around sipping beer/wine in the corner while the kids go on the rampage out of sight for you, I'm afraid).

Our armoury includes:

• Medication pack.
• Wet wipes for mopping up spills/cleaning hands (anyone's) and wiping surfaces.
• Safe snacks – where possible to match what the party host is providing. If not, then some favourite treats so your child doesn't feel they are missing out.
• Party plate, paraphernalia and favourite drinking cup or bottle – we've learned from bitter experience that being the only kid without a Ninjago paper napkin can be a devastating affair.
• Extra treats, edible or otherwise, for unexpected happenings – the piñata nobody mentioned, or the pass-the-parcel prize your little one can't eat. When our son was small we would stash a secret Lego minipack in our bags in case something cropped up requiring emergency action!

Wipes yes, gels no

When wiping hands and surfaces, use wet wipes or carry a pack of reusable clean cloths and a portable spray dispenser of detergent and water. Remember, liquid hand sanitizers and gels do NOT remove allergens. They kill bacteria and viruses but simply smear food proteins about. You don't need to use special antibacterial or sterilizing wipes – studies have shown that any wet wipe or cleaning product will do the job.

What if our allergen is on the menu?

If there's something on the menu that you're worried about – hummus, say, or Nutella sandwiches – think through the risks and see if you can mitigate them.

Could you make a polite request that all the children wash their hands after eating, or use wet wipes? Could your child be popped on an end seat so you can keep an extra eye? If it seems like a big risk, talk it through with the host and see if you can come up with a plan, or adapt one or two things. There may be times when you feel the risk is genuinely too high – a baking party, for example, with lots of very small and rambunctious kids, or a restaurant that you don't feel happy about.

It's obviously easier to politely decline an invitation when your child is too small to realize they've even been invited. Then again, when they are bigger there will be less random food-hurling and your child will be better able to manage risk themselves.

'We've said no thank you to a pizza decorating party in a place we knew wasn't geared up to deal with allergies, and only gone to half a party – the cinema bit but not the restaurant bit.'

'Every toddler party we ever went to served ice cream and we just had to manage it. We were always there keeping a close eye, and aside from one or two itchy rashes he was fine.'

'We've been lucky – at all the parties we've been to the parent has asked if there's anything really bad for us that they should exclude, so we always vetoed sesame or nut anything. We had to take the risk with being around cheese sandwiches. It's a balance of what's reasonable and what you can cope with.'

'We've been to plenty of parties with pizza served for all the other kids, but we brought our own milk-free food and I watched him like a hawk!'

'I've had fantastic experiences with some party venues, for instance subbing a slushy for ice cream for my daughter, or checking every ingredient for me.'

'I stayed at parties until he was at least ten. After that, we started with parents I knew very well and showed them how to use his meds. I totally sat in a restaurant near the party, though ... she texted to say they were heading home and we had to fling ourselves in the car to be back before her!'

How to deal with tricky family or friends

With family, or close friends, it ought to be different. You would hope that they would make adjustments to keep your child's allergens away, or safely out of reach. We have an unwritten rule, which is that family events are always safe for our son. He is never going to be fully included in other events, so we figure let's have one safe space where he knows he will always be able to eat everything that's on offer.

I appreciate that, unfortunately, not all families are as understanding. Or not every member of your family will be understanding. A soft start might be to point them at one of the allergy resources at the back of this book. Education and awareness can help, when simple lack of info is the problem.

There comes a point, though, where you do have to put your own child's happiness and safety first. If a family member or friend repeatedly ignores your child's allergies or creates a situation that is potentially unsafe or genuinely upsetting, it may be that you've just got to say 'no' the next time.

Here are some experiences and solutions that fellow allergy parents have shared with me:

'We eat before we visit, take our own food when we go, and just ignore the gibberish some people spout.'

'We've had this a lot – "can't she eat a Snickers bar?" Or, "it's only a bit". We eat before we arrive or take our own food. There's

no other way. Some people aren't interested in understanding, others have got better but it's never 100 per cent safe with them. And the rest are brilliant, so it's a mixed bag.'

'Sadly, I found sharing news reports of tragic incidents the most useful strategy to get people to take allergies seriously. Not in the presence of the person with the allergy, obviously.'

'We've tried to teach some people but they either didn't get it or thought we were too extreme. We had some near-misses and so decided to take the extra anxiety away. It can be tough, but it was just too stressful.'

'Worst was one relative who bluntly asked for written evidence that the allergies were real! He just couldn't believe we had two children with allergies.'

'Early on, we bought and sent our closest family a book about childhood allergies – we realized there was a lot for the whole family to learn.'

'We've never expected special treatment, but several people have surprised us and gone the extra mile, which is lovely. There are very kind and thoughtful people out there so do take heart, even if you're going through a tough time with some friends or family right now!'

Ten ways to throw an allergy-friendly party

If you're looking to host a party for someone else with allergies, or to give a friend or family member some top tips, here are a few ideas to share:

1　Fill piñatas with non-food surprises – small toys, mini rubbers, bouncy balls, hair slides ...
2　Instead of a sweetie-stuffed party bag, what about a book, a pair of novelty socks, a diary and pen, or a Lego minifigure? Some companies sell children's books at a discount in collections of ten or 20. Or you can buy assorted Lego minifigures in bulk from eBay; divide the heads, bodies, accessories etc.

into different pots and let the kids build their own character to take home.

3 Consider non-food prizes for party games, or having a suitable allergy-friendly alternative so nobody is left out.

4 Dole out snack food like popcorn or crisps in individual bags to avoid cross contamination ...

5 ... and pick common snacks (e.g. crisps, raisins or popcorn) that don't contain major allergens such as milk, wheat, soya, egg, nuts, sesame, and don't have 'may contain traces'. Instant easy inclusion!

6 Prep a few simple items, such as cucumber sticks or fruit kebabs, on clean equipment away from all other foods, and pack a portion in a sealed container for the child with allergies to have. Don't forget clean hands!

7 Some foods can easily be adapted to make them allergy-friendly for all – you could sub a dairy-free spread for butter in ham sandwiches, for example (check all labels first to make sure the bread and filling don't contain the allergen either).

8 Reassure the allergy family by checking all packaging and labels with them in advance – send pics or ask about 'safe' brands they use. Where possible, keep their child's food in the original closed packet for extra reassurance.

9 Ask if there is a safe treat you can buy to give the child when the cake is being doled out.

10 Let the allergy parent help. They will often feel a bit like a helicopter parent, and someone who's bulldozed the run-up to your party with questions and demands – so help them feel useful by asking if they would like to help hand out the food on the day. That way they can also keep an eye on proceedings without feeling awkward.

Bake sales

Bake sales are always going to be a bit dispiriting, there's no getting around it. Some days it just feels too sad having to hustle your little one past trestle tables piled high with cookies and cakes, friends clamouring around clutching coins in one fist and a tower of napkin-bundled brownies in the others.

But there are ways to help your child feel included and raise a little bit of awareness, too.

Bake safe

When I have the energy, I bake safe cookies or cupcakes and label them as 'nut, egg and sesame free'. I keep aside a few in a Tupperware for my son, and hand over the rest in a sealed box. People see that allergy-friendly food can look and taste nice (imagine that!), and my son has something that other kids are buying from the stall. I started on a performative mum mission baking elaborate Cookie Monster cupcakes and all sorts, not least to prove that allergy doesn't mean you can't have the best cakes on the block. But that became a bit high intensity, so I just make something that looks generally pretty these days.

Bake really safe

When I've really had the energy (rare), I've even packaged the cakes and cookies in individual sealed bags and added my name and phone number, so any passing allergy family can ring me to check whether I know what I'm doing!

Buy and donate

Some bake sales can be militant about 'homemade only' but there's a good argument for buying packets of allergy-friendly treats and donating those, too – that way anyone with allergies has access to the package labelling. If I'm honest I probably wouldn't buy anything homemade from a bake sale for my son, even if it was individually packaged with the parent's phone number on it! Also, providing pre-packaged treats raises awareness among others that there are brands out there that might be good for those with allergies. AND my son can buy one straight off the stall like any other kid. Even sealed individual bags of popcorn are a treat.

Some more points to consider:

If your school/nursery is a nut-free setting, then you are perfectly within your rights to insist a bake sale is too – allowing nutty cakes would (a) send mixed messages and (b) pose something of a risk. Bake sales are not policed in the way school lunches are, so food gets everywhere. I do think asking for a bake sale – or a school – to be free from 'may contains' is an ask too far.

I got a little exasperated when I first started helping out with our school PTA and saw 'not suitable for allergy' and 'may contain nuts' signs plastered all over the place at the first sign of any fun. So I made sure that any event I was involved in had some sort of allergy-safe option, and replaced those signs with ones that read something like:

'All food is homemade or provided by parents/carers and many will contain allergens or have been made in an environment where allergens are present. BUT we often have allergy-friendly options, so please ask stall-holders.'

It's worth noting that school bake sales (ditto church bake sales, charity fundraisers etc.) class as 'occasional, small-scale' events so aren't subject to allergen labelling laws. If the food is provided on a 'regular and ongoing basis' one would need to register as a food business anyway, and that's when statutory allergen information should be provided.

Here are some other ways parents have managed bake sales:

'I make my son's 'safe' cake and take it in. He buys his cake back, which is kept in his Tupperware on the bake sale table, clearly labelled. Sometimes I make a big one so others are able to eat what he is eating.'

'Whatever we donate, I keep some aside and then bring it along to the event.'

'I try to carry homemade equivalents in my bag (the mental load of this sort of thing is a whole other story!).'

'I man the stall with the safe option in Tupperware and hand it directly to my son!'

'We donate nut and peanut-safe homemade cakes – marked up as such – but keep some at home for my child so we know they're not contaminated.'

'If I'm not there, I give my daughter her own box of goodies and make a separate donation to the sale.'

'We got involved. A group of fellow allergy parents wrote guidance and patrolled a special allergy table!'

'I took in a cupcake and the teacher gave it to my son in nursery. He felt included with everyone else. Such a happy smile on his face!'

How to handle playdates

Unfortunately, your child probably won't want you tagging along to his mate's house to play on the Xbox when he's 13. Outrageous, I know.

The truth is, play dates can be nerve-wracking. All you want is for your child to be 'normal' and to socialize with their friends. So getting an invitation to play is a double-edged sword for any allergy parent – joyful, but also the trigger for a lot of anxiety and worry.

While your child is young it's pretty straightforward. You go with. Or, you find a trusted and understanding parent and train them on how to use your child's AAI, what your child's allergy symptoms are, what risks to look out for and perhaps also provide your own snacks and food.

Here's a checklist for training a fellow parent:

- Send them a video of how to use your child's AAI – the Anaphylaxis Campaign has good online resources, and the individual device manufacturers may also have videos and info to download.
- Consider asking them to complete some online allergy awareness training – the Anaphylaxis Campaign has a set of free resources for parents and carers at <allergywise.org.uk>. They will need to commit to about 45 minutes online for this!
- Provide them with an AAI trainer pen – again, the manufacturers have these available to order online.
- Sit with them and go through how to use your child's AAI device, including asking them to demonstrate.
- Give them a printed copy of your child's BSACI Allergy Action Plan, which explains the key symptoms and how to treat them.
- Show them your child's personal medication kit and what's in it.
- If they want to cater, and you feel comfortable with this, suggest something very simple – a safe pizza, for example, or ready meal that can be popped straight into the oven on a foil-covered tray and served up without any additions or amendments.
- Provide a pack of safe drinks and snacks and/or a list of ones they can safely buy.
- Tell them you're happy to check any ingredients or packaging any time.
- Tell them you're equally happy for your child to ring you if they have any anxieties while they are there – explain

that they may need reassurance from you to begin with, especially around food.

- Tell them you'll be in the shed at the bottom of their garden for the duration of the play date.

OK, I'm (half) joking with this last one, but don't think yourself alone if you decide you need to position yourself nearby when your child first ventures out without you. A cup of tea in a nearby café, sitting in the car working on your laptop, having a stroll in a nearby park: if it helps you make that transition, do it. But remember this is only for the first couple of occasions. Your child enjoying a play date without you means a little free time for you, after constant 24/7 vigilance for so long.

If it all feels too much, clinical psychologist Dr Mary Halsey advises starting to look for manageable opportunities first. 'Go to a family event and allow your child to play in another room with other children for a bit. Go easy on yourself and acknowledge it is a hard thing to do because, for so long, you as a parent have been the one to make sure your child is safe. If your child is on a play date without you and your instinct is to phone every half an hour, maybe allow yourself to phone once. Prepare yourself and your child by having a conversation now and again – "what would you do if this happened?" Allow them to start asking their own questions, or do a few things for themselves, so you can see if they are OK – and if they are not then it just needs a bit more work.'

Clubs and activities

When other parents grumble about the slog from sports club to dance class, swimming lesson to art session, I confess inside I am screaming – just a tiny bit – 'TRY STICKING AROUND FOR THE WHOLE HOUR AND A HALF OF EVERY SESSION, EVERY WEEK, EVERY MONTH, FOREVER.'

OK, I exaggerate. But while other kids casually get dropped at ballet, or football, and mum or dad nip off to have a coffee, get some work done, or just go home, I'm usually still sitting there, like a giant lemon, playing with my phone on a wobbly child-sized chair in a drafty corridor.

I have to confess I haven't often left my son alone when he's had any out-of-school clubs. Either the teacher hasn't ever had EpiPen training, or they feel happier if I'm on hand, or I can't face the rigmarole of going through everything yet again and it seems easier to spend a mindless hour and a half sending dog GIFs on WhatsApp. As he's got older, though, I know it's a step we need to take. It helps that with age comes greater awareness, so he knows not to eat food that hasn't been supplied by me and, generally, the clubs he takes part in don't have any food involved anyway.

The first thing to do is ask: many formal activities, especially those run by bigger organisations, have EpiPen and anaphylaxis training built into their First Aid. For example, Girlguiding and The Scout Association 1st Response First Aid training covers anaphylaxis, as do FA coaching emergency aid courses. If not, a coach or teacher may be willing to undertake some training – depending on the situation, you might give them a lesson yourself, as you would with another parent, or recommend a First Aid course. Alternatively, the Anaphylaxis Campaign has free courses for carers of pre-school and school-age children at <allergywise.org.uk>.

If snacks or refreshments are offered, the easiest thing is either to recommend or provide safe snacks for everyone – or send your child with his or her own pack of food and drink.

12

Must-have recipes

Every allergy family has one – the failsafe recipe you just can't do without. Here are a few that have got us through:

Absolutely the best cake recipe ever

I cannot even begin to say how easy and amazing this allergy-safe cake recipe is. As usual, I left it until the last minute to get prepping for my son's third birthday (how clearly I remember, the year before, pledging to perfect all manner of sweet treats by the time he turned three. Ha!) and, in a state of panic, tweeted my worries about finding the right recipe. Back came a link to something called 'Wacky Cake', an American concoction apparently created during the Depression era when fresh ingredients were rationed. It contains no egg, no dairy, no nuts and can be baked with gluten-free flour, too. It uses vinegar or lemon to replace the egg – and it works.

Suddenly I had a pile of perfectly pretty, firm and fluffy looking cupcakes ready for icing. I had chocolate ones, vanilla ones, lemon ones …

So, I am eternally grateful to my Twitter friend and fellow allergy parent Kate for this. She said it would be a life changer and it is.

Ingredients

225 g self-raising flour

or

265 g gluten free flour plus 1 teaspoon xanthan gum

225 g caster sugar
1 teaspoon baking powder
(*optional 3 or 4 tablespoons cocoa powder*)
½ teaspoon salt
1 tablespoon white wine or cider vinegar
5 tablespoons sunflower or rapeseed oil
½–1 teaspoon vanilla essence to taste
240 ml warm water

other options include:
Vanilla cake: omit the cocoa and double the vanilla extract
Lemon cake: omit the cocoa and substitute lemon juice for vinegar,
adding lemon zest to taste
Orange cake: omit the cocoa and substitute orange juice for water

Method

1 Preheat oven to 175°C non-fan.
2 Mix the dry ingredients together thoroughly.
3 Mix the wet ingredients together separately, stir to combine.
   When using lemon, pour the lemon juice in last.
4 Add the wet ingredients to the dry, mix to a smooth batter
   (but do not beat).
5 Pour into a greased and floured 9″ round or 8″ square cake
   tin, or 12 cupcakes (top tip: using a silicone baking 'tin'
   reportedly makes a big cake less crispy).
6 Bake the full cake for 35 minutes and cupcakes for around
   20 minutes, or until firm to the touch and a skewer comes
   out clean.
7 Decorate as desired!

Absolutely the second best cake recipe ever

There are lots of vegan recipes out there subbing yoghurt for
egg, but this one appeals because there's minimal faff and

straightforward ingredients. For chocolate cakes I always revert to the 'Wacky' version (above) but for a simple vanilla or lemon I think this is my favourite. It's always moist and delicious, and has a lovely rise. You can use dairy or alternative yoghurt. I find it needs a good glug more liquid than the recipe allows, so I usually add a liberal dash of milk to smooth the batter out, but other than that it never fails me.

Ingredients

200 g self-raising flour
100 g caster sugar
2 teaspoons baking powder
150 ml yoghurt or soya yoghurt
5 tablespoons sunflower oil
1 teaspoon vanilla essence

Factor in some extra liquid depending how runny your yoghurt is – you may need to add a dash of milk or milk substitute to loosen out the cake mix at the end. You can replace the vanilla with lemon juice and zest.

Method

1 Preheat oven to 180°C.
2 Grease and lightly flour 1 x 10″ cake tin.
3 Sift dry ingredients – flour, baking powder and sugar – together.
4 In a separate bowl mix the yoghurt, oil and vanilla essence.
5 Combine the two mixtures and beat for a minute with a spoon.
6 Pour into the tin and bake for 20 minutes or until risen and golden on top.
7 Remove from oven and allow to cool, before turning on to a wire rack.

Pancake Day saviours

Shrove Tuesday is another date in the calendar that poses challenges to those of us with egg, milk or wheat allergies. This vegan, fluffy American pancake recipe is great for a stack of blueberry-topped fat ones.

Ingredients

125 g self-raising flour
2 tablespoons caster sugar
1 teaspoon baking powder
Pinch of salt
150 ml milk (dairy free or otherwise)
¼ teaspoon vanilla extract
4 teaspoons sunflower oil

Optional: switch the vanilla for one small mashed banana and/or a scattering of blueberries stirred into the mix.

Method

1 Sieve the flour, sugar, baking powder and salt together in a bowl and mix well.
2 Add the milk and vanilla (or banana) and whisk to a smooth batter. If adding blueberries, stir these in after you've whisked.
3 Wipe some of the oil around a large non-stick frying pan and heat. Test with a drop of batter – if it instantly bubbles up, you're good to go.
4 Pour in around two tablespoons of pancake batter and turn the heat down. Use the back of a spoon to spread the batter into a 10–15cm circle. Add more batter to create a second pancake, and if your pan is big enough, a third.
5 Cook until bubbles are popping on the top of the batter and the edges start to look a little drier. Flip over and cook on the other side for around a minute – you're looking for golden brown, so keep an eye on the heat.

6 Keep the pancakes warm, placed individually rather than in a pile on a baking sheet in a low temperature oven until you're ready to serve them all up.

Here's a recipe for a more traditional British crepe-style pancake. This one was given to me by an Instagram friend, Nia. As an EpiPen-carrying woman who is 'allergic to lots', she is an expert on all things allergy friendly, from doughnuts to biscuits and, yes, pancakes.

I honestly couldn't tell the difference between these, doused with a little lemon and honey, and their egg counterparts. You can make them gluten free by simply substituting in gluten-free flour; ditto dairy free by switching for a milk substitute. I think they might be just as good with a savoury filling.

Ingredients

200 g self-raising flour
250 ml milk or milk substitute
150 ml water
2 tablespoons pure sunflower oil

Method

1 Sieve flour into bowl and pour in milk or milk substitute, water and oil.
2 Mix well with balloon whisk, fork or spoon.
3 Wipe a non-stick pan with pure sunflower oil and heat.
4 Ladle mix into the pan and 'swill' to cover base thinly.
5 Cook, flip, cook and eat!

Easy free-from Christmas Pudding

Another seasonal staple that's hard to find if you're avoiding more than one allergen. This recipe is gluten, dairy, egg and nut free and makes a two-pint pud – enough for a family of ten to have a decent slice each.

Ingredients

100 g gluten-free bread flour
100 g soft brown sugar
2 teaspoons mixed spice
50 g prunes
50 g dried apricots
125 g sultanas
125 g raisins
125 g currants
50 g mixed peel
50 g glace cherries
1 orange – juice and grated zest
1 lemon – juice and grated zest
50 g sunflower oil

Method

1 Sieve the flour, sugar and mixed spice together and stir in a large bowl.
2 Chop the large dried fruit in a separate bowl – big chunks or small, however you prefer them – and mix with the rest of the dried and candied fruit.
3 Add the lemon and orange zest and juice, along with the oil. Stir together.
4 Add in the dry ingredients and stir well.
5 Cover the bowl with a tea towel and leave for at least two hours, or overnight.
6 Prepare the basin by oiling the inside of it. Cut two circles of greaseproof paper to fit just inside the top. Pour the pudding mixture into the bowl, pushing it well down and smoothing over the top. Pop the greaseproof sheets on top.

7 Cover the top of the basin with foil, securing it tightly around the outer rim by tucking in or tying with string.

8 Put the pudding in a large pan with boiling water halfway up the basin.

9 Simmer for two hours with the lid on, adding extra boiling water as it evaporates (don't forget to keep checking!).

10 Remove from the pan and leave to cool, keeping the foil on top.

11 Keep it in a cool dark place for four to six weeks.

12 On the day, replace both the foil and greaseproof paper circles with fresh ones.

13 Simmer as per step eight for one hour. Remove the pudding and serve!

Aeroplane breakfast bars

I always struggled with a travel-friendly breakfast for early airport trips and flights. This is actually a baby weaning recipe someone gave me, but for a few years (once we'd outgrown the banana allergy) it worked as a portable, filling breakfast-on-the-go. It's just little fingers of oats and dried fruit, but you could scatter in anything really – safe seeds, chocolate chips, freeze-dried berries ...

Ingredients

One ripe mashed banana
5-6 tablespoons rolled oats
2 tablespoons plain flour
2 tablespoons small or chopped dried fruit (sultanas, apricots etc)

Method

1 Preheat the oven to 180°C.

2 Stir the oats and dried fruit into the mashed banana – you want to create a fairly pliable 'dough' that can be shaped with your hands, so not too sticky. Add a little flour until you achieve the texture you need.
3 Shape the mixture into 'bars', and place on a lightly-oiled baking sheet.
4 Bake for ten to 15 minutes until lightly golden.
5 Cool and serve. Can be frozen.

All-you-ever-need quick soft cookies

These 14-allergens-free soft cookies crop up on my fellow allergy mum friend Laurna's Instagram page in all manner of wonderful guises – pink and swirly, sandwiched with raspberry 'cream'; plump vanilla mouthfuls dotted with rainbow sprinkles; cocoa-rich mounds of melt-in-the-mouth biscuit-ness. She says: 'As an allergy parent all you really need is one basic soft cookie recipe and about three different cutters. You just pimp them up from there.'

Make these chocolate by adding a tablespoon of cocoa; add Sunbutter for 'nuttiness' or 100s and 1000s for prettiness; make two flavours and pipe them together if you're feeling really flash; sandwich them with dairy free 'butter' icing; add a spot of colour to the mix to brighten up a rainy Wednesday. The cookie is your oyster. You can find more of Laurna's recipes at <myallergyboy.com>.

Ingredients

¾ cup gluten-free self-raising flour (make sure it contains xantham gum)
¼ cup caster sugar
¼ cup dairy-free margarine
1 tablespoon golden syrup
1 tablespoon rice milk

(Optional: 2 heaped tablespoons dairy-free chocolate chips)

Method

1 Preheat oven to 190°C.
2 Line baking tray with greaseproof paper.
3 Mix sugar and marg well together, then add golden syrup and rice milk and stir well.
4 Add the flour and mix until combined.
5 Stir in the chocolate chips (or whatever else you fancy).
6 Use a teaspoon to scoop, and another to push the mix on to the baking tray – leave space between as they spread in the oven.
7 Bake for ten minutes. Cool. Eat.

Lucy Parr's dairy-free summer berry fro-yo

This quick and easy dairy-free frozen 'yoghurt' recipe is courtesy of the amazing Lucy Parr of <lucysfriendlyfoods.com>. She is a Cordon Bleu-trained chef and mum to two children with allergies to milk, egg, sesame and nuts.

Her blog is packed full of gorgeous vegetarian recipes, from allergy-friendly doughnuts to egg-free meringue, so do check it out for inspiration.

She describes this simple three-ingredient 'fro-yo' as 'light, refreshing, yet creamy and utterly delicious'. It also takes only minutes to prep and a couple of hours to freeze. You can sub in any frozen fruit you fancy.

Ingredients

250 g frozen berries
2–4 tablespoons icing sugar
1 tablespoon water
250 g dairy-free yoghurt, ideally Greek style

Method

1 Use a food processor or high speed blender to blitz together the frozen berries, icing sugar and water. You will end up with a granular paste.
2 Add the Greek-style yoghurt and whizz until smooth.
3 Freeze for an hour.
4 Stir and then freeze for another hour. Easy!

Substituting egg

- *If you want to substitute one egg in baking, add 1 teaspoon of baking powder; OR 1 teaspoon of bicarbonate of soda plus 1 teaspoon of lemon juice.*
- *To replace one egg for binding, use 1 tablespoon ground flaxseed/ linseed mixed with 3 tablespoons water (leave to stand for ten minutes before using); OR sub in 2 tablespoons of sunflower oil.*
- *Gram or chickpea flour can make a good 'eggy' sub for the real thing when whipping up an egg-free omelette, vegan French toast or a no-egg quiche. There are lots of vegan recipe ideas online.*
- *Bird's custard is egg free – it was invented in 1837 by Alfred Bird, whose wife had an egg allergy!*

Find more substitutions in this handy guide from allergyadventures.com:<http://allergyadventures.com/media/43915/Allergy_ Substitutions.pdf>.

Egg-free meringue miracle

Aquafaba. If you haven't yet heard of this chickpea/bean juice miracle, I suppose you've been doing more exciting things than experimenting with the dregs of a legume can.

Originating in the online vegan community, the use of aquafaba – the gloopy brine water you get in a tin of white beans or chickpeas – has revolutionized the world of egg-free baking. It can be put to use in a multitude of ways, from fluffy mousse to Yorkshire Puddings. And it creates a really stunningly impressive meringue. Here's Lucy Parr's own take, from her blog <lucysfriendlyfoods.com>:

Ingredients

1 tin of chickpeas or white beans

½ cup caster sugar plus 3 tablespoons set aside, both whizzed in a blender to become finer; OR you can use icing sugar (as long as it doesn't contain any cornflour)

¼ teaspoons xanthan gum

1 teaspoon vanilla extract (or flavouring of your choice)

Method

1 Drain the chickpeas, letting the liquid fall into a large bowl – and set the pulses aside for another day.

2 Add the xanthan gum and whisk on high speed until the mixture forms soft, billowy clouds.

3 Add the sugar, 1 tablespoon at a time, letting it mix fully between each spoonful.

4 Once all the sugar is incorporated, whisk in the vanilla (or other flavouring).

5 By now you should have stiff peaks of meringue fluff.

6 Pipe or spoon on to lined baking sheets – try making small ploppy 'kisses'.

7 Bake at 120°C for 30 minutes.

8 Turn the oven down to 90°C and cook for a further 1 hour.

9 Turn off the oven and leave to cool for another hour.

10 Now you can eat, dip in chocolate, sandwich together with your choice of cream or use to decorate a cake. Keep in an airtight, dry container – but bear in mind these will only stay fresh for a day or two.

Top baking tips from allergy parents

'Best baking advice I ever got was that regular biscuit recipes work well even when you're swapping out ingredients. Dairy-free spread for butter, gluten-free flour for wheat flour. A biscuit recipe is pretty much a biscuit recipe.'

'Icing sugar mixed with dairy-free spread on a plain biscuit is a proper treat. Add a little cocoa and it's a chocolatey treat.'

'Freeze cookie dough in a sausage shape, and you can just slice off a chunk, defrost and bake.'

'Biscuits freeze and can be eaten pretty much straight out of the freezer.'

'Keep a stash of safe treats in the freezer for emergencies – a few cupcakes, a scone or two, some cookies, some uncooked sausage rolls. Then even an eleventh-hour party won't faze you.'

'Make egg/dairy/gluten-free breaded chicken, or fish goujons, by dipping in whichever safe yoghurt you can use, followed by your choice of safe crumb.'

(See 'Resources' at the back for some allergy-friendly cooking blogs.)

13

Starting nursery

Gulp. The big step.

My husband and I are self-employed, so we decided that, between us, we could just about juggle enough to defer nursery until our son was three. I was so nervous about sending him off and wanted to wait until he could communicate how he felt. I appreciate that is a luxury not everyone can manage. There are obviously options outside of a nursery or playgroup setting – family, a child minder, a nanny, and those choices are very personal ones that depend on circumstance and more. In this chapter, however, I'll try to cover the checks and steps you should follow when choosing and starting nursery, and then school.

We began our search pretty early. There are crazy waiting lists in our area (I'd heard of otherwise sane parents putting their impending babies' names down the minute the stick turned blue) so we checked out the local options about a year ahead of time. I'd recommend this regardless, as it may take time to find the setting you are most comfortable with.

We had heard good things about the nearby community nursery, set in a Victorian former fire station, with its philosophy of celebrating diversity, representing a proper cross-section of local people, all that fine stuff. We booked ourselves in for an open day. It was a bit hectic and tumbledown but had a nice feel and the kids looked happy. So I asked: 'What's your policy on children with severe food allergies?' 'Oh, it's no problem,' came the answer. 'We've got loads of kids who are vegetarian, and even one who doesn't like cheese.' You might say she was the wrong person to ask – she wasn't the manager, just one of the nursery assistants – but, for me, unless every single member of staff, permanent or itinerant, is properly trained in food allergy control and EpiPen use, it's out of the equation.

Another nursery, in a terraced house on the street next to ours, had seemed so promising. Then the manager told us how she had the kids baking croissants every week. When I asked how she might be able to accommodate our son and his allergies, she looked at us sternly: 'I suppose he can put them in bags when they're baked.'

After some trawling about, we found a nursery that seemed to have its act together. It was cosy, jammed with cushions and squashy dens and books, and immaculately clean. As parent to an allergic child it's the first thing you look for – in doctors' waiting rooms, playgroups, cafés, even (guiltily) other people's houses: how clean is the floor, how clean are the toys? More often than not there are crumbs coagulating in the corners, smears of food, smudgy fingerprints. For most parents this would be fine: a little bit of dirt's got to be good for the immune system, right? But for us it's a gateway to worry: were those mucky hands clutching a peanut butter sandwich? Are those crumbs from a seed-packed breakfast bar? Is that smear – yikes – hummus? But the joy of this nursery was that, peer as I might (and I can peer mighty well), everything looked spotless, spick and span. On the walls were boldly printed, meticulously typed sheets detailing the various allergies of children at the group – this one's coeliac diet, that toddler's milk allergy. In the kitchens the prep areas were carefully delineated and potential allergens kept at a safe distance from foods eaten by allergic tots. A member of staff was charged with monitoring each child with an allergy during every mealtime. They were EpiPen trained at regular intervals – and given booster training every time a new allergic kid was admitted. Hurrah. We put his name down.

Key things to think about

Do they have an allergy policy, and any other children with allergies?

This isn't a deal-breaker, but it helps if they have a system in place. More important than this, though, is whether or not you get the sense they are listening, empathetic and willing to adapt to accommodate your child.

Big warning signals are the blithe and breezy 'don't worry about it, we've got it covered' alongside a reluctance to go into details. This would worry me just as much as a place that seemed clueless or unwilling. Look for somewhere, and someone, that is happy to give the time to chat and go through your questions and concerns. Even if they haven't got all the systems, if they are happy to work with you that's so important.

Are staff regularly EpiPen trained?

Not only do you need all staff responsible for your child to be trained in how to deal with an allergic reaction, there needs to be regular refresher training. Before your child starts, you want to hear that they are all having a booster session, and that they ideally retrain everyone annually. A community allergy nurse or your paediatric allergy clinic should be able to help if training is required.

How do they manage food on-site?

Whether or not your child will be staying for meals, you need to know how the nursery handles food and drink on-site.

Questions include:

- How does snack time work? Do they help themselves, or are they served?
- Do kids have direct access to jugs and beakers of milk?
- How would staff adapt to make sure there is no chance of

your child coming into accidental contact with his or her allergen?

- Do they check for 'may contain' info with their suppliers?
- Are families allowed to bring food on site (e.g. for birthdays)?
- How do they handle special occasions or cooking activities?

We provided our son's morning snacks, approved by the nursery, and any fruit was prepared and served to him separately from the other kids. We also sent him in with a clearly-labelled water bottle (his photo laminated and attached to the neck by an elastic band) that was kept out of reach of other children to avoid anyone accidentally taking a swig.

When we plucked up the courage to let him eat lunch, we approved every meal in advance and checked ingredients with the chef. His food was served by his key worker only, on a red plate to mark it out from the other meals. Another option is to provide a safe packed lunch for your child each day. It absolutely has to be a personal decision by the family, so go with whatever suits you best.

'The nursery cook provided lunches for our daughter, who has allergies to egg, nuts, sesame and milk. I think it's completely doable and a potentially important opportunity for allergy kids to have a chance to eat out of the home regularly, with peers and without lots of drama. It allows them to build trust and confidence in others and it supports families because it gives them a break. BUT it requires planning and commitment from kitchen staff, catering companies and nurseries or schools. Training and communication is key.' – Kate, allergy parent

Food bans

I talk a bit more about nut bans in the 'schools' section, where it becomes more relevant (see Chapter 14). In an early years setting it is highly likely that nuts wouldn't be permitted anyway, as they pose a choking risk, and I think there is a strong argument for peanuts and tree nuts to be vetoed among pre-schoolers. Sesame bans may be similarly enforced. These are foods that can easily be removed from menus and activities.

It gets trickier when you come to food that is a 'staple' – milk or wheat, say, or egg. Here, a ban isn't necessarily feasible or achievable, so it comes down to the systems the setting has in place to manage risk. Nuts, peanuts and sesame were banned from the nursery we chose and I'll confess it absolutely did give me peace of mind. Our other allergens, such as egg, weren't, but the chef and staff had clear systems in place to ensure no cross contamination.

This is a discussion to have with your nursery or playgroup. You need to have a clear sense from the school that, if your child's allergens are allowed on-site, they are managed incredibly carefully with your child always in mind. For example, if one child has a milk allergy, having open jugs available for the others to help themselves would pose a significant risk. An alternative could be for staff to pour milk, given to the children in a specified area, and for tables, chairs, mouths and hands to be given a wipe down afterwards.

Provide an Allergy Action Plan

The British Society for Allergy and Clinical Immunology (BSACI) provides an Allergy Action Plan template which can be personalized for your child. Your allergy clinic should provide you with one of these – or contact your GP for them to complete one for you. The draft template can be viewed online at <bsaci.org/professional-resources/resources/paediatric-allergy-action-plans/>.

The plan lists your child's name and allergies, with a space for his or her photo and date of birth. It outlines how to use their AAI (there are different versions depending on what device he or she is prescribed), and common symptoms to look out for.

It also details the dosage of antihistamine in the event of a mild reaction. This document should be updated every year under the guidance of your allergy specialist or GP.

We have always requested that these plans are not only kept on file in nursery and school, but displayed in prominent locations for easy staff access – and as a constant visual reminder. Our son's plan was on display in the kitchen, the staff room and the nursery room he was in. Another copy was kept with his medication.

Create an individual risk management plan

Every child, and every allergy, is different. Nobody knows how your child reacts better than you, and all of that information will help your child's teacher or key worker to care for them. I have always typed and printed out a personalized 'risk' plan – key bullet points outlining:

- Which allergens to avoid
- What symptoms to look out for
- Where risks may be (mealtimes, soap when washing hands, messy play, trips, drinking water) and how to mitigate them
- Any other information such as allergies to plasters, hay fever, eczema, asthma and so on.

There are examples of detailed risk management plans in the schools section.

Keep medication within safe reach

Medication should be kept in a clearly-labelled box, with your child's photo and name on it, in easy reach and access of all staff – but out of the reach of children. It should not be locked away in an office, but always on hand for immediate use. Make sure you and the nursery keep note of the expiry dates and these are replenished in plenty of time.

Make sure all staff and families are aware

If other families are allowed to bring food on site, check that the nursery will inform everyone that there is a new child with allergies, and caution against anything that might pose a genuine risk.

Sometimes children may be allowed to bring in treats for birthdays and other celebrations. There are two ways to deal with this – one is to ask that food is not permitted to be brought in from home, but that you and the nursery work together to find a suitable treat for all. Or you provide a list of safe treats (or even an emergency bag of non-perishable safe treats) for your child to have in this event, so long as serving and eating the birthday food is done safely and with no risk of cross contact. Inclusion is key here: it's not OK for your child to be sat alone while the other kids tuck into Colin the Caterpillar.

No sharing

A 'no sharing' policy is an important rule to instil, so that all children are aware that they cannot share food or drink. It's also something to keep reminding your child about – never to take food that is offered by anyone other than the approved staff. The staff should be aware that your child may question if food is safe, so they need to explain that they have checked the item with you and give reassurance. They should never dismiss an allergic child's concerns over food without a proper explanation to reassure them. If your child is very anxious, it is reasonable for them to call you so you can speak to them.

What if your key worker is away?

There should be a system in place should your child's regular key worker be absent or sick, to ensure that he or she always has someone with them who is aware of their full allergy history and is trained in use of an AAI.

Baking, messy play and crafts

This is another question to raise early on – how will they ensure there are no risks from junk modelling or other craft and food activities? A solution is to ensure no food packaging is donated by families, or none that might include traces of allergens such as nutty breakfast cereal boxes or egg cartons.

If your child is allergic to certain foods, ensure none of these are used in sensory play – e.g. dried pasta or lentils – and that any food to be handled is completely free from your child's allergens and not to be consumed.

Baking is possible, with a bit of forethought. For example, on Pancake Day our son's nursery had all the children making egg-free pancakes. When they had a little summer party to celebrate 'graduation', the chef made an egg-free cake for all. The key here is regular communication and for both parties to be willing to pitch in and help with ideas and resources.

Give thought to any art materials – some modelling clays contain wheat, and some paints (albeit rarely) contain egg. Face paints are another thing to watch out for – but there are allergy-friendly options available, so research these first (see Chapter 21). Similarly check for latex in equipment such as aprons, rubbers and so on. Growing cress in eggshells would be another cause for concern, as would the shared use of wind instruments – consider having a clean, unused one set aside solely for your child's use.

Wheat-free modelling clay recipe

Ingredients

140 g rice flour
60 g cornflour

    2 tablespoons cream of tartar
    170 g table salt
    1 tablespoon oil
    240 ml cold water
    Food colouring (your choice!)

Method

1 Put all ingredients in a saucepan – aside from the colouring – and stir well with a wooden spoon.
2 Heat over a low heat, stirring continuously, until the mixture 'clumps' into a dough. This should only take a few minutes.
3 Turn the dough out on to a board or worktop covered in greaseproof paper, and let cool for a minute or two, then knead until smooth. If it is sticky, add a little more cornflour.
4 Divide into balls, indent the top of each with your finger and pop a little food colouring into the hole. Knead – and go!

Cloud dough

As the name suggests, cloud dough has a lovely soft feel and is great for sensory play for little ones. It's not sturdy like modelling dough, but lots of fun to mess around with.

Ingredients

    1 kg bag of rice flour
    250 ml vegetable oil

Method

1 Mix or rub together in a big bowl until the oil is completely integrated into the flour.
2 Place in a high-sided tray container and add scoopers and pots.
3 Let them dig in with their hands.

Animals

If animals or birds are on-site, or visits are arranged, check the feed for potential allergens. Look for bird feeders in outside play areas – peanuts and sesame may be commonly included.

Trips and visits

Your child should always have an EpiPen-trained member of staff with them on trips, and consideration should be given to any food that might be needed. We would give our son's key worker a pack of wipes to clean down any chairs and tables if the kids were going to be eating packed lunches away from the nursery. If there are visits from entertainers or educators, these people should also be reminded about allergies and not to include food or risky modelling materials.

Handwashing

Simple, but key. Instilling regular handwashing avoids the risk of contaminated little hands. Remind the nursery that soap and water are needed rather than sanitizing gels or sprays – the latter don't get rid of allergenic proteins. Soap is best – although check for allergens, such as milk or nuts – and in the absence of that, a scrub with a wet wipe. It's a good idea to have children wash their hands on arrival, and then before and after eating food. Toilet goes without saying!

Extra resources

Allergy UK and the Anaphylaxis Campaign have great resources for parents and childcare settings. Visit their websites for videos, info packs and downloadable documents.

You can check your childcare setting's latest Ofsted inspection report via <www.gov.uk/ofsted>.

There are some really nice downloadable packs too from <allergyadventures.com>.

What does the law say?

The Statutory Framework for the Early Years Foundation Stage can be found on the Department for Education website. It sets out the standards for learning, development and care for children from birth to five, given legal force by the Childcare Act 2006. It covers all early years providers, in the state and independent sectors, as well as daycare, childminders and nannies on the Early Years Register or registered with an early years childminding agency. It states the importance of 'equality of opportunity and anti-discriminatory practice, ensuring that every child is included and supported'. It also notes that 'providers must take all necessary steps to keep children safe and well' (Section 3.2). They must have a policy for administering medicines, including systems for obtaining information about a child's medicines, and keeping that information up-to-date. Training 'must be provided for staff where the administration of medicine requires medical or technical knowledge'. Providers must also keep a written record each time a medicine is administered and inform the child's parents and/or carers 'on the same day, or as soon as reasonably practicable'.

With regards to catering, before a child is admitted the provider has a duty to obtain information about food allergies and 'providers must record and act on information from parents and carers about a child's dietary needs'. They must be 'confident that those responsible for preparing and handling food are competent to do so' and all staff involved in the preparation or handling of food must have food hygiene training. They must also undertake thorough risk assessments and 'be able to demonstrate how they are managing risks'.

What if something isn't right?

What should you do if your childcare setting is not putting the right systems in place, or is ignoring your child's needs? All registered childminders, daycare providers, nurseries, playgroups and pre-school settings must – by law – have a process for handling complaints. See <www.gov.uk/complain-about-childcare> for more information.

The first step is to speak to your child's key worker and the setting manager. If you agree steps to resolve the issue, follow up via email so the action is there in writing. It may also be useful to give the nursery allergy information videos and fact sheets to share among staff, as these resources can add further weight and knowledge.

You could also ask your allergy clinic if one of their nurses can help. Dr Mary Halsey, clinical psychologist for allergy at Southampton Children's Hospital, says: 'Our specialist nurses sometimes have conversations with schools or nurseries if there are big problems. The key thing is really good communication and often it takes more than one conversation to understand allergies. They may not have had experience of allergies before.'

If you are still facing problems, you may wish to escalate to the setting owner. All providers must investigate written complaints relating to their fulfilment of the Early Years Foundation Stage requirements and notify complainants of the outcome of the investigation within 28 days of having received the complaint. If you think your child is at risk, contact your local council. By the time it gets to this stage, obviously many will have decided to remove their child. However, if you think the issue may be discrimination because of your child's healthcare needs, you could contact the Equality Advisory and Support Service for guidance via <www.equalityadvisoryservice.com/app/ask>.

Ofsted is the place to go for complaints about the setting as a whole – although they cannot consider individual issues or investigate specific incidents. You must also have first followed the school's complaints procedure. If they do decide to carry out an inspection you won't be informed of it directly – those results will be published online.

14

Starting school

If I had to give just one piece of advice on dealing with allergies in school it would be: communicate. Keeping lines of communication open between you and the school is fundamental to a good system, and a good relationship.

Sometimes you will feel like 'that' helicopter parent, always mithering the teachers with questions about EpiPens and lunchtime supervisors. Be bold and do it – never be too afraid to ask, or to clarify. At the same time, make sure the school knows you are happy to help in any way at all, be it providing safe resources, on-the-hop advice, or talking through ideas to make a science experiment or cooking session safer.

The steps to finding the right school aren't too dissimilar to the steps to finding the right nursery. Look at Ofsted inspections online, ask friends in the area. Book in a few visits and ask to speak directly to the headteacher and/or the health and inclusion lead. This may be the SENCO (Special Educational Needs Coordinator), but all schools have slightly different set-ups so there may instead be a lead admin for health, or an on-site school nurse. Find out who takes responsibility for managing children with medical conditions and ask to speak to them directly.

Will my child get priority admission to my chosen school because of his/her allergies?
In general, conditions including allergies, asthma, eczema and diabetes are not among the medical conditions given priority for admissions. This is because they should be able to be supported in all mainstream schools.

You will need to check with your local authority but, generally speaking, if you feel your child's condition merits special consideration you need to demonstrate how this has a significant impact on your child, and why a particular school can meet their needs more than another. You will also need to supply a statement from your GP or doctor.

Checklist for starting school

Individual Healthcare Plan (IHP)

This is a statutory document provided by the local authority and the school, which you will fill out before your child starts. It should be updated at least annually by the school nurse or appointed member of staff. All pupils with medical conditions – including food allergies – should have an Individual Healthcare Plan agreed between the parents and the school. This is particularly important where an adrenaline auto-injector (AAI) has been prescribed for use in emergencies.

It is worth noting (but don't let this scare you) that teachers and other non-healthcare professionals are permitted – but not obligated – to administer an AAI. We have, over the years, been asked to sign a standard disclaimer within our Individual Healthcare Plan that states: 'I understand that the school is not obliged to give medication'. Other parents I know have been presented with plans that include the statement: 'We cannot guarantee medicine will be given'. As a rule I always cross that line out and initial my amendment. It's never come back to me yet.

As well as information on your child's condition, their symptoms and emergency treatment, an Individual Healthcare Plan should consider dietary requirements and issues such as travel on school transport – who is responsible for the medication – and so on.

Unfortunately, the level of detail in most IHPs is, to be honest, substandard. Ideally, it should also include every element of risk management, from lunch to PE to details of what training has been given to whom. Have a look at the Health Conditions in Schools Alliance website at <medical-conditionsatschool.org.uk> for a great example of the perfect IHP template. However, most school plans currently aren't detailed enough to cover all bases, so I – like a lot of fellow allergy parents – create an additional 'allergy risk management' document. Coming up next ...

Allergy Risk Management Plan template

To supplement the basics in his Individual Healthcare Plan, I rewrite my son's personalized allergy plan every year when he starts with a new teacher. As we've moved on from Reception it's become less detailed as the school has developed a good system and he becomes more aware of the risks himself.

The first plan I wrote was pretty full-on, but I stand by that – to begin with, as long as it's clear and doesn't place undue demands on the school, the more information the better. Nobody's ever told me to get lost, anyway, so I keep on handing it out: a copy for the new teacher, one for the SENCO, an extra one for the files. When my son started school, I met with his new Reception teacher, the SENCO and the school nurse at the end of the preceding summer term. The plan I then wrote was really just a documented record of everything we had discussed and agreed.

Here's a version of our own Reception plan, which might be handy as a springboard for your own.

[Child's Name] - Allergy Risk Management Plan   [Date]

With any queries/concerns at any time – even if just a quick check – please contact child's parent/guardian on [telephone number].

Bob is severely allergic to:
EGGS
PEANUTS
TREE NUTS (i.e. all other nuts such as cashews, Brazils etc.)
SESAME
LENTILS

He can react on contact to these foods and carries two EpiPens and cetirizine antihistamine (the latter only for mild, localized reactions, e.g. a few hives on the skin). Full treatment procedures are outlined in his BSACI allergy action plan, to be displayed with his photo in class/lunch hall/other public areas as necessary.

The key thing is that any accidental contact is avoided.

LUNCH
Bob will start reception having packed lunch but may move to school lunches, in which case this plan will be revised and updated. The key points at lunch are:

- Table and chair to be clean of any food residue/traces.
- Bob to wash his hands with soap and water before eating.
- Bob will need close supervision during lunch times, not only to help him build confidence to know what he can and can't eat (e.g. if his food falls on the floor or on another child's plate he can't then pick it up and eat it due to the contamination risks) but also to ensure nobody else's food has contact with him, or his meal.
- It would help greatly if the other children are aware that Bob can't ever share food/cups/cutlery and that they have to be careful not to touch his food/him while eating – and the reasons for this (i.e. Bob is allergic to some foods and they can make him ill).
- Encourage classmates to wash their hands after mealtimes.
- Sanitizing liquid does not remove allergens – it 'smears' the allergic proteins around – so a good wash with soap and water or, at the very least, a thorough clean with a wet wipe is needed.
- Parents to provide Bob's water in a bottle flask, clearly labelled. This water is for his use both in class and at lunchtime.
- Spare 'emergency food' bag to be kept in class, in the event of Bob dropping his lunchbox/his lunch becoming contaminated. Parents to replace the food items each half term.

- Consider Bob's location in the lunch hall – would it work for him to be at the end of a table or in the same place so lunchtime supervisors are always aware?

SNACKTIMES/FOOD IN CLASS
Bob is fine with fresh fruit but it's important that the food he eats isn't handled by other children, also that anyone preparing this fruit washes hands beforehand. For any other snacks (e.g. raisins) please check with parents first as some brands are 'safe', others are not.

Teacher A has suggested Bob might have the task of carrying the tray out and taking the first piece of fruit. Or his fruit could simply be given to him first. It's important that there is never any accidental sharing of food, so close supervision will be needed to ensure the fruit isn't put down/absent-mindedly picked up by the wrong person. If necessary, a plate should be provided for Bob. If other children also have plates, Bob's should be clearly differentiated either by labelling or by colour etc. Parents happy to supply if needed.

If there is any other situation where food is eaten/brought into class, please try to give parents at least a week's advance so they can check any 'may contains' issues with the manufacturer or come up with a safe alternative. Sometimes manufacturers can take a while to respond, or 'safe' versions can be hard to get hold of, which is why advance notice would be really helpful.

COOKING IN CLASS
Please discuss in advance. Parents are very happy to help with safe options, and also to provide an easily available list of 'safe' ingredients (e.g. flours, as some are processed on the same lines as sesame seeded flours; or icing sugar, as some may contain egg).

EQUIPMENT IN CLASS
Junk modelling, sensory play, craft with food etc. should all be checked – no lentils, no boxes that previously contained nuts/sesame and no egg cartons. Modelling clay/flour etc. to be checked for allergens (most are fine). Any tempera paints to be checked as a minority are egg-based. Any wind instruments (e.g. recorders) to be thoroughly washed with washing up liquid and water before Bob uses them. Any pasta for play to be egg free.

EPIPENS

Bob's parents will provide two EpiPens and his antihistamine with syringe in an insulated, labelled bag (EpiPens have to be kept at an even temperature, so not left on a radiator, for example). The medicine bag must go wherever Bob goes – in class, outside for break, in the lunch hall, fire drills, on trips. Named adult to be responsible for carrying Bob's medication and returning it to its place in the classroom; a second adult to be allocated as a 'deputy' if needed. Bob to be made aware of which adult has his medication and who to approach if he feels he may be having a reaction. When Bob is dropped at school his parents will also leave his second 'travel' kit of medication in class and collect it with him at the end of the day. Parents have responsibility for checking medication is in date and replacing it when needed.

TRIPS

Please meet with parents when any trips are planned to go over potential risks.

SOAPS, LOTIONS

Please check any soaps for staff/children don't contain sesame (*Sesamum indicum*) or any nut oils/milks.

SUPPLY STAFF/LUNCHROOM SUPERVISORS/VISITING TEACHERS

All staff, including temporary or lunchtime staff, to be made fully aware of Bob's allergies and of the need to avoid any contact with his allergens.

Tracey Dunn, headteacher at Fitzmaurice Primary School in Wiltshire, has created a standard Allergy Risk Management form, which is now widely used across Wiltshire and is available via the Anaphylaxis Campaign website. There is a downloadable version at <https://www.anaphylaxis.org.uk/campaigning/making-schools-safer-project/> which you may wish to plunder.

Allergy Action Plan

As with nursery, I provide the school with the BSACI paediatric Allergy Plan (see Chapter 13) that details his allergies, what symptoms to look out for and how to treat an allergic reaction. I give several copies for the files and also to be displayed with his photo in the staff room, lunch hall, classroom and medical room.

When General Data Protection Regulation (GDPR) regulations on data privacy came in, we had a very minor tussle over whether the plan could continue to be displayed in public. I sought advice from the Anaphylaxis Campaign and also the Information Commissioner's Office (<ico.org.uk/>). They state that there are three areas where you can justifiably keep these posters on display. The first is very simply consent – so with the consent of a parent it is absolutely fine, as long as you document that consent. The other two, in the absence of consent, may be 'legitimate interests' and 'public task' and the info relating to these is here: <https://www.gov.uk/government/publications/supporting-pupils-at-school-with-medical-conditions--3>

The school has been happy with me confirming my consent via email.

What are schools obliged to provide?

Schools have a legal duty to make arrangements for pupils with medical conditions (including those with food allergies). In England this sits under the Children and Families Act 2014.

In each of the UK regions the law is supported by statutory guidance: in England this is 'Supporting pupils at school with medical conditions', which you can find at <gov.uk>. In Scotland it is 'Supporting children and young people with healthcare needs'; in Wales it is 'Supporting Learners with Healthcare Needs' and in Northern Ireland it is 'Support for Pupils with Medication Needs'. The legislation applies to state schools, academies, free schools and pupil referral units. It also 'applies to activities taking place off-site as part of normal educational activities'.

Independent schools are subject to the Schedule to the Education (Independent School Standards) Regulations 2014. This states that schools should 'have proper policies' to protect the health, safety and welfare of pupils, but you will need to discuss your individual school's allergy policy with the school leadership. For specifics you should refer to the relevant documents listed above, although all four UK nations remain broadly in line.

In general, the statutory guidance says all pupils with medical conditions should be properly supported to have full access to education, including school trips and sports. The English guidance notes they should be able to 'access and enjoy the same opportunities at school as any other child'.

Governing bodies must ensure that systems are in place and appropriate healthcare professionals are consulted where necessary, and also take account of the needs of each individual child. The guidance adds: 'It is ... important that parents feel confident that schools will provide effective support for their child's medical condition and that pupils feel safe.'

No child with a medical condition should be denied admission or prevented from taking up a school place because arrangements for their medical condition have not been made. An eye should be given to the potential for bullying, or a child's anxiety, depression or self-consciousness around their condition.

School policies should also aim to:

- determine who is responsible for ensuring all staff are adequately trained;
- ensure all relevant staff will be made aware of the child's condition;
- make sure there is cover in the event of staff absence or new staff;

- brief supply teachers;
- conduct risk assessments for school visits, trips and other activities outside of the normal timetable;
- monitor and regularly review individual healthcare plans.

There should be procedures in place to cover transition between schools, or the need to update a pupil's plan if their circumstance changes.

All schools also have obligations under the Equality Act 2010. Where severe allergy can be said to constitute a physical impairment that has a substantial and long-term effect on a person's ability to carry out day-to-day duties, it would be considered a disability under that Act. For example, in 2013 an employment tribunal (Wheeldon v Marstons) ruled that a chef's severe nut allergy qualified as a disability requiring his employers to make 'reasonable adjustments' to accommodate his needs.

'The Equality Act is very important and I think perhaps under-utilized by the allergy community. It's particularly relevant with regards to adjustments in schools. It's not a blank sheet for everything to be made allergy safe – adjustments must be reasonable – but it's really useful for supporting arguments that schools think through activities and find ways to make them inclusive. It basically applies to every situation where an allergy parent thinks, 'If you had just told me you were doing X or Y activity I could have explained to you how you could replace Item A with Item B and the activity would have been safe and accessible for all the kids'. It's really important for inclusion. For example, having the allergic kid separate and on their own isn't OK. Even if you call it the 'sunshine table' as one school we visited did.' – Kate, lawyer and allergy parent

Spare pens in schools

Since October 2017, all UK primary and secondary schools can buy AAIs from a pharmacy without prescription for use in emergencies on children at risk of anaphylaxis, but whose AAI is not available, or not working. However, these devices should be considered only as a back-up device and not as a replacement for the child's own AAI. The parent would have to provide written consent for use of the spare in the event of an emergency, usually in the Individual Healthcare Plan. It is also only permitted to be used on children deemed medically 'at risk' of anaphylaxis – although they won't necessarily have had to be prescribed an AAI. More information is available at <sparepensinschools.uk>.

What's missing?

While the statutory framework is important, many doctors, parents and campaigners still feel there is not enough accountability built into the school system to ensure every setting complies. For example, they argue that medical conditions need to be seen as part of the rigorous safeguarding policy and practice – which currently they are not. And they would like to see very specific allergy and anaphylaxis policies written into law.

In a 2020 editorial[1] in *Clinical and Experimental Allergy*, the official journal of the British Society of Allergy and Clinical Immunology, paediatric allergy consultants Dr Paul Turner and Professor Adam Fox joined Anaphylaxis Campaign chief executive Lynne Regent and Allergy UK chief Carla Jones in demanding 'urgent action' around schools. They said the current statutory framework was 'wholly generic' and did not

---

1 'Keeping food allergic children safe in our schools – time for urgent action', Turner et al, *Clinical & Experimental Allergy*, 2020. See: <https://onlinelibrary.wiley.com/doi/full/10.1111/cea.13567>

provide detail about specific medical conditions. They added: 'Consequently, schools must develop their own food allergy policies, from scratch. This inevitably leads to inconsistency: there are examples of excellent practice, but we frequently hear about schools where the opposite is true.' Where high-profile incidents have happened, very often poor staff training is at fault. They call for funding for anaphylaxis training in schools, as well as making it a legal requirement to introduce measures to minimize risk, and to ensure all staff understand which children are at risk and why. The authors add: 'The most successful approaches have utilized a 'whole school' approach, where policies are developed in partnership with parents, pupils and healthcare professionals and involve 'whole school' education – pupils, teaching and non-teaching staff alike.'

The Anaphylaxis Campaign has developed a Making Schools Safer[2] online resource to help parents and schools improve allergy provision (find it at <anaphylaxis.org.uk>). Its chief executive Lynne Regent says: 'All staff regardless of role should be trained in allergy and anaphylaxis. At the moment, the statutory framework is guidance so there is no legal expectation for schools to comply. And the current Ofsted Inspection framework doesn't have a focus on children with allergies.'

If allergy were to be included in safeguarding legislation – 'Keeping Children Safe in Education' – failure to comply with procedures could lead to a no-notice inspection or even closure of a school. Local Authorities and Academies would have a duty to ensure that its schools are compliant.

The little-known Health Conditions at School Alliance, whose members include charities, healthcare professionals and trade unions, also want:

---

2 Anaphylaxis Campaign: Making Schools Safer Project 2021: <https://www.anaphylaxis.org.uk/campaigning/making-schools-safer-project/>

- Ofsted to tell their inspectors to routinely check schools' medical conditions policies as part of their regular inspections.
- The Department for Education to change their guidance, so that all schools need to publish their medical conditions policies on their websites.
- The Department for Education to do more to help schools understand their responsibilities and put together quality medical conditions policies.

They have a range of resources to help schools at <medicalconditionsatschool.org.uk>.

A headteacher's eye view

'One of the hardest things I navigate, as a head, is ensuring that I meet the needs of all my pupils. While I have children with allergies, I am also balancing the needs of children who are diabetic, asthmatic, epileptic and many other conditions. As a parent, I truly only appreciate the needs of my own child and I have to fight for my child, this is the same for every parent. School has to balance all these needs so that children are not at detriment because of another and all are safe.

I often feel that parents expect schools to be experts in managing allergies and sometimes have unrealistic expectations of what is practical to achieve. I feel that anxiety often gets in the way of good working relationships.

I advocate for and believe that schools need to be allergy aware with a high level of knowledge and training; with systems and processes that keep children safe. They also need strong relationships with parents where staff don't feel like they are being judged for asking questions.

Parents should expect that:
- schools are not necessarily experts in allergy management. They may never have had any experience with allergies and they genuinely may suggest what seem to be 'silly things' (to an allergy parent) because they are rapidly learning and genuinely don't understand;
- statutory guidance is implemented;

- there is a robust policy for managing medical conditions which explicitly includes allergy;
- the child is fully included;
- key staff are trained;
- there are good relationships with key staff where both parties can have productive communication and neither side feels a nuisance to the other;
- the school will listen to the parent;
- there is accountability for keeping the child safe through the school's policies - for example, through the complaints process which already has to be published on the school website.'

– Tracey Dunn, primary school head and parent to a child with allergies

Catering

As with all food prep businesses, school caterers are subject to the EU regulations on labelling, which came into effect in December 2014. Staff must be aware of these rules – including the fact that they have to declare whether their dishes contain any of the 'Top 14' allergens as an ingredient. Kitchen staff must be able to easily identify those with specific dietary requirements. This could be by displaying a photograph of the child alongside details of their allergy in the kitchen and/or serving area; or the use of a coloured wristband to identify those with dietary needs.

Catering for allergy comes under the same guidance as outlined in the sections above – whereby schools have a duty to support pupils with medical conditions. In England, for instance, the Standards for School Food say dietary needs should be catered for – including 'pupils who cannot eat certain ingredients due to an allergy'. Even if meals need to be adapted at short notice, those pupils' needs should still be met.

Anecdotally, the provision across the UK is hugely patchy – some schools handle catering for allergy brilliantly. Others dole out jacket potatoes five days a week, while some school caterers even put a 'cap' on the number of allergies per child they will accommodate. This is clearly unacceptable.

Meet with your school catering manager and go through your needs and concerns in detail. They should not only make reasonable adjustments to cater for your child, but also provide a healthy variety of options through the week.

A parent's eye view

'One of the key things is to be clear who is responsible for overseeing catering and who can serve as a point of contact. In our case it was the SENCO who coordinated meetings between us, the catering company and the cook. We used to go through the menu each term and identify which meals were suitable.

I think, as allergy parents, we also have to recognize the immense pressure that the cooks feel and be reasonable. They are cooking for many kids, on tight budgets and sometimes in pretty cramped kitchens. I was always extremely grateful for their willingness to undertake the extra work. If they said something wasn't possible then I accepted it. I also accepted that the substitutions would be imperfect, in terms of a totally balanced diet, and sometimes the meal would be repetitive, but the goal was finding a way to allow my child to eat safely outside of the home and learn to trust other people to manage her dietary needs outside of her family.

It was also important to have a designated person – a lunchtime monitor – who was responsible for overseeing that the right food was received. This person was also the person that my child could speak to if they weren't sure or they weren't feeling well.

You need to expressly explain that your child cannot eat X or Y allergen or anything which contains it as an ingredient or a trace. I cannot begin to tell you know many conversations I've had where I've had to say, "no, she can't have quiche, she's allergic to egg" and the person has said, "wow, never really thought about it, so can she have cake?" "No. No she can't if it contains egg". And repeat.

You need to talk about label checking. You need to talk about cross contamination. We used to ask for her food to be cooked separately and then wrapped in clingfilm with her name on it and served to her that way. This provided reassurance. It also avoided the risk of cross contamination in the hectic time of food service. It also was useful when she was younger because she knew only to eat the food that had been covered and named as being for her.'

– Kate, whose daughter, 11, is allergic to egg, nuts, sesame and milk

Other school issues

Complaints

If you are unhappy with an area of your child's allergy care, the very first step is to speak to the health lead, such as the SENCO, the school head or your child's teacher. More often than not, issues can be resolved with an informal meeting and by talking through concerns.

We've had situations that have briefly upset me – finding out there were freshly cracked eggshells in class ready for a science experiment, for one, and the time my son ended up in 'after school club' without anyone who knew he carried an EpiPen. But these were isolated incidents that came from either good intentions or accidental oversights – luckily no harm came from them, and the situations were quickly remedied ensuring they didn't crop up again. In fact, they ended up being 'learning opportunities', which ensured any loopholes were closed and extra checks put in place.

If you aren't happy with the response, however, your school's governing body will set out how complaints should be handled and you should make a formal complaint via this procedure. If you still have no success then, depending on where you are in the UK, there are various next steps. In England, you can make a complaint to the Department for Education under certain circumstances – ensuring all other attempts at resolution have been exhausted first. In Scotland, there is the option of a local authority process, third party mediation or an Education Appeals Tribunal.

You can take independent legal advice, and also seek help or advice from the allergy charities. Both the Anaphylaxis Campaign and Allergy UK run helplines (see back of book for resources) and their staff are well trained to advise on common issues affecting families of children with allergies.

Remember it's not 'one size fits all'

This one bears repeating on a few counts. So, even if your school has had, or currently has, other children with allergies and systems in place to deal with those allergies, it doesn't mean their systems will automatically be right for you.

Every child has different allergies, and differing needs. Severity and type of food hypersensitivity will vary, and some parents may well be less strict about things like 'may contains' and so on.

We certainly found that, although there had been other kids with EpiPens in school, the school didn't have a standard system for starting school other than the local authority-devised IHP. This document didn't cover the mitigation of risk or where it might be good to adapt systems and processes (for example, how to deal with lunchtimes, travel and so on). We were also told that we were more 'strict' about food than other parents. It's tricky when this happens, because you always run the risk of being painted as the overprotective parent, but frankly I don't care. We're vigilant at home and I expect the school to be equally vigilant when my son is in their care. What other parents do is irrelevant.

It's worth noting that the government guidance for England, 'Supporting pupils at school with medical conditions', advises that it is not acceptable practice to 'assume that every child with the same condition requires the same treatment'.

The other way in which it's not 'one size fits all' is in how each school differs physically and logistically. Ours is a single-storey 1960s building sprawling across a fairly large footprint – so keeping our son's EpiPen in class as he moves around the place isn't ideal. Other schools will differ in their geography – if it's a small village school, keeping AAI pens in one place may make more sense (just not in a locked place). The key is to talk these specific requirements through and come to a plan that suits your circumstances.

Your role

As parent or carer you are responsible for providing the school with sufficient and up-to-date information. You should be involved in the development and review of your child's healthcare plan, and make sure that you provide medicines and replace them when expired. You should also provide contact details for you, and/or another responsible adult, to be contactable at all times. Under government guidance, medication kept in school must be in date, labelled, in the original container and include instructions for administration, dosage and storage.

After a reaction

If at any point your child requires their medication in school – including antihistamine – your school should follow the allergy action plan. It is the school's responsibility to keep a written record of all medicines administered, and parents should be informed.

If your child needs to be taken to hospital, staff should stay with them until a parent arrives, or accompany a child to hospital by ambulance. A school should not send a child who has become unwell to a school office or medical room unaccompanied, or with someone unsuitable. If a reaction occurs in school, there should be a meeting or discussion between the school and family about what happened, and how future risks may be better mitigated.

School trips

Your child's medical needs should not prevent them from participating in school trips, visits or sports activities. Reasonable adjustments must be made to accommodate them where necessary.

A risk assessment should be carried out before any trip or visit, in consultation with the family and pupils. And a school should not place obstacles before participation by 'requiring' a parent to accompany the child if this is not possible or reasonable.

After school clubs

These vary, with some schools offering clubs and activities led by staff, and others recruiting outside companies to take classes. In primary, you would expect someone who is EpiPen trained to be with your child.

Our school has been great with clubs – there are several EpiPen-trained Teaching Assistants (TAs) on staff, and one of them always accompanies our son to club. We organize this termly with the lead for after school enrichment, and I keep in regular touch with her via email. If the session leader is from an external organization, I usually also arrange to have an in-person chat before the first club takes place, and talk through our son's allergies.

The school has a 'no treats' policy anyway, although we have fallen foul once – a well-meaning teacher in gardening club brought chocolate coins for the class at Christmas. Luckily, my son refused, having had the 'don't accept food from other people' rule hammered home until his poor ears bled. The school made sure to reiterate the 'no treats' rule more stridently after that.

We had one slip-up, where the usual TA was off sick and nobody was allocated in her place, so my son toddled off to club without his EpiPen or anyone who was aware of his allergies. He came to no harm but it jogged both me and the school to put extra checks in place – his teacher supervises handover of my son and his medication to a named person, and I check in with the after school enrichment lead via email every week or two to make sure his usual TA is there.

Absences

Government guidance states that a school should not 'penalize children for their attendance record if their absences are related to their medical condition, e.g. hospital appointments'.

It's a big bugbear of many allergy parents – well, many parents of children with all manner of medical conditions – that 100 per cent attendance is often rewarded by schools with treats or certificates. If your child finds this unfair or upsetting, it may be worth having a chat with his or her teacher to point out that the absence isn't avoidable and shouldn't be indirectly punished.

Treat box

Provide a pack of emergency non-perishable foods – a 'treat box' – to be kept in school for your child in the event of emergencies. It can cover any eventualities, such as a hiccup in your child's lunch (think trays being upended on the floor ...) and also unexpected 'treats' – for instance if there's a popcorn and movie afternoon, or a class birthday. I usually include things with a shelf life to last half a term: sealed packs of crackers, dried fruit, popcorn, oat bars, favourite biscuits.

Nut bans

This is a tricky one. There are arguments for and against banning specific foods from schools and nurseries. The arguments for are clear – remove or at least minimize risk, raise awareness by letting others know about allergies, and allay allergy families' anxiety. On the other hand, there is an argument that banning certain foods might encourage complacency: 'there are no nuts here, so we're allergy safe'.

The allergy charity the Anaphylaxis Campaign is generally not supportive of blanket bans of allergens, saying: 'This is because peanuts and tree nuts are only two of many allergens that could affect pupils, and no school could guarantee a truly allergen-free environment for a child living with food allergy. We advocate instead for schools to adopt a culture of allergy awareness and education.' But they do point out that schools have a 'duty of care', and decisions should be made around specific children's needs. They add: 'In nurseries and infant classes, it is reasonable to ask parents not to allow children to take peanuts and tree nuts into school, in order to reduce the risks of cross contamination for particularly young and vulnerable children. Schools caring for older children should undertake a thorough risk assessment and may wish to write to parents asking for their cooperation in making life safer for the children in their care.'

In practice, what does an allergen ban mean? Are all foods with 'may contain' labels banned too? Do you ban any allergen a child might have? Milk? Wheat? Strawberries? Can you be sure that every parent bringing food into the setting has remembered or understood the ban? Is banning food enough? Might it mean that allergy protocols become less strict, or rigorous, if the setting assumes everything on-site is 'safe'?

As mentioned in the nursery section, I'm largely in favour of minimizing risk as much as possible in any early years setting – and arguably in primary. Our primary school has a nut and sesame ban, which is a mixed bag. It means parents are periodically reminded not to pack those foods in their children's lunches, and I know they aren't on the school menu, either. But, of course, parents don't fully understand what this means, so I'm pretty sure foods like pesto, Bakewell tarts and nutty snack bars make it through the school gates. Egg – sandwiches, quiches, mayo – are all used, so of course the environment isn't risk-free.

Unless it poses a direct risk, I tend to focus on how the school is managing crunch points like lunchtimes, so my son stays safe. Systems to look for include:

- Making sure tables and chairs are clean, or your child gets to sit at an unused table.
- Check that your child is still able to sit with friends – there is no good reason to place 'allergy kids' on one table away from their peers.
- Ensuring lunchtime supervisors know about your child's allergies, are EpiPen trained and his or her med kit is within easy reach.
- Lunchtime supervisors should be primed to keep an eye out for any food-related incidents around your child.
- Handwashing before eating is important – I never completely trusted that my son washed his hands before lunch, so I pack wet wipes in his lunchbox with strict instructions to give his hands a scrub before tucking in.
- In an ideal world, children would also wash their hands after lunch.
- Strict 'no sharing' rules should be enforced.

Food in class

This is one of those things you should discuss in full with your child's teacher before they start a new year. Schools have wildly differing policies on food treats in class.

One of the reasons we chose our local primary is because they had a 'no treats for birthdays' rule already in place. It's not as mean as it sounds – but it did mitigate the risk from cakes and cookies arriving from children's homes. Parents were allowed to take in fruit kebabs, or popcorn. I remember painstakingly drawing funny faces in marker pen on satsumas to take in for his 30-odd classmates on his birthday. Where a child in class had a specific fruit allergy, these were vetoed. This is where the emergency food bag comes into play – I wouldn't let my son eat food prepped by other people, so he'd fish out a safe pack of popcorn for himself. Non-food treats is another option – stickers, or pencils – although thought should be given to non-food allergies such as latex, too.

Class parties are another crunch point – make sure your teacher knows to pre-warn you if they are planning any kind of food activity. Talk through safe options, and you can either provide a safe pack for your child to eat, or sealed packs for his exclusive use. Remember to talk through science experiments and cookery, too: with preparation all of these things can be made safe, but the key – as always – is communication.

Involve your child

As your child gets older and heads towards secondary school – say, Year 5 or 6 – it is a good idea to involve them in any Individual Healthcare Plan or allergy care document. They should know where their medicine is at all times, and be helped to be confident enough to speak out if they are worried about food, or feel they may be having a reaction. If your child is nervous or shy, or unwilling to put themselves forward, it may be worth having a chat with their teacher so they can reassure them that it is the right thing to speak up.

It's also helpful to introduce your child to self-carrying their medication on a step-by-step basis – you know best what your child can take responsibility for. A good first step might be for them to carry their medication into class and hand it over every morning, and then – under teacher supervision – to carry it between lessons or to after school clubs. The aim would be for your child to be able to self-carry by the end of primary school. If your child is too anxious or unwilling, they should not be forced by the school. The family and school should discuss together the best course of action.

15

Transition to secondary school

And then all of a sudden your wobbly toddler is striding off to secondary school in massive shoes. The idea is enough to frighten any allergy parent – primary school, in comparison, seems a cosseted and cocooned environment. How will your child cope with self-carrying their medication 24/7, navigating the chaos of a secondary school canteen, the fear of bullying, the peer pressure. Actually, more to the point – how will you cope?

In the next chapter, I cover the steps to helping your child become more independent around their allergies. But here are some tips on how to handle the logistics of starting secondary school.

What to look for in a secondary school

- Before making your selection, speak to the person in each school responsible for medical conditions – this will vary, and may be a nurse, administrator, SENCO or pastoral lead.
- Ask what their processes are for managing children with allergies – who is EpiPen trained, which staff are responsible, where is spare medication kept, how do they manage trips and food-related activities, do they have other children with allergies in school?
- Ask whether there will be one main point of contact both for you, and your child, should there be any concerns about allergy issues.

- Who will be responsible for contacting you if there are any queries (for example, around food-related activities, or school visits)?
- Ask how they share information on children with allergies across the school – how do they ensure that all your child's teachers will be aware, including potential supply teachers?

How to prepare for Year 7

Ahead of your child starting, make sure you:

- Email the school to give them full details of your child's allergies, including their allergy action plan and a risk assessment similar to the one outlined above for primary.
- Arrange a meeting with your child's form tutor, head of year and/or the person in charge of medical conditions to discuss your child's allergies, EpiPen training, school trips, food related activities and catering and so on – you can do this in exactly the same way as you did for primary school.
- Train your child in how to administer and carry their own EpiPens, and pick out an insulated med bag they are happy with (see Chapter 16 for ideas).
- Although your child will now self-carry, make sure the school also keeps a spare set of two adrenaline devices for your child in an accessible place – probably a medical room – together with his or her BSACI allergy action plan and any other spare medication (antihistamine, inhalers).
- Check the 'chain of contact' – secondary schools vary and you will need to know who your child's main point of contact is if they have any concerns about allergies in school, and who your contact is, too.
- Consider lunches – will your child take a packed lunch? If not, arrange to speak to the catering manager and talk through the options.

- Try to speak with or meet the head of Home Economics before term starts, so that they have time to plan for inclusion.

'I know my son's risk assessment is logged on the school information management system and that all the teachers are able to see this. He has had the same tutor throughout, and she is really good at getting in touch with me when needed – especially around things like treats. I've cultivated my relationship with both her and the student receptionist. She is simply lovely and in the first year she would often phone me to say, "do you think he is worried about x, y or z?" Now he doesn't go to her at all.

With things like trips, or PE competitions, or cooking, I would get in touch with the relevant subject lead directly. I find myself having to be a bit more proactive but that's fine.

It's really important that children are prepared to manage their allergy for themselves as they move through school. In Year 7 they have a huge responsibility and if their parent has always managed it for them (and the school has always been allergen free), it doesn't equip them to be confident in managing their allergies for themselves.

We do a huge amount of scenario-based coaching to equip him with the skills he needs. There have been times when I have quietly had a word with school without my son knowing because of an incident that has happened. He very much does not want me interfering and he also does not want the world to bend to accommodate him; he feels that this will single him out and make him a target for bullying. Whether or not this is accurate or would happen, we don't know. But young people need to have their voice heard and be respected.' – Tracey Dunn, primary head and allergy parent

'Be prepared to make face-to-face appointments with heads/ department heads/school nurses, as that has more impact on their understanding of severity of the allergies. Keep that connection going via email and phone calls. Things may go wrong, but you will have

that connection to work with and get changes or support put in place.'
– Sarah Chapman, allergy parent

Sarah Leggatt's son is 18 and has multiple allergies:

'To be honest, I have found secondary schools in general to be better at dealing with allergies than primary. They seem to have more experience of the issues involved.

We taught our son to self-administer his EpiPen when he was nine, so he was well prepared to self-carry by the time he started secondary. I also taught his best friend how to administer his EpiPen, much to my son's annoyance! He practised self-carrying his EpiPens the year before he started secondary to get used to carrying them in his bag.

At the start of year 7, the school arranged an overnight trip to a Viking educational centre. The idea was to live as a Viking for 24 hours, including making Viking food! The aim of the trip was to bond with their tutor group, form tutor and head of year. My son rarely did overnight school trips in primary. The school discouraged my son from going after reading his allergy plan but he really wanted to go, so I visited the centre in person and talked to the amazingly helpful course leader. She went through all the food and said he could bring his own cereal for breakfast. I wrote up my own risk assessment for the trip (four typed pages of A4!) before the school was happy to take him. All went well, except he came back wheezing. They spent the night sleeping on stone benches in front of a fire. The fumes got to his chest. I was so focused on the food, I forgot about his asthma!

He has done plenty of day trips, including in sixth form, to academic conferences in London. On the last trip he ate a packed lunch in McDonald's while everyone else tucked into their burgers and chips. I'm more bothered by this than him.

Other food issues: there are unfortunately similar issues to primary with teachers giving students sweets as rewards. Food tech was a challenge in Years 7 and 8, but he adapted recipes and had a safe space far away from the others.

For his food allergies generally, I liaised with his form tutor, head of year and the amazing office team leader. Before any school trips, I'd always call her and she'd confirm that an EpiPen-trained staff member would accompany the trip and that his emergency medicine box would be taken, in addition to the one he carries in his bag.'

Trust your judgment

If a school doesn't feel right – even after you've gone through the whole application process – don't be scared to make a move. One parent reveals how she switched her choice at the last minute over allergy concerns:

'We actually ended up at a school completely different to the ones we applied for. We got third choice and when we started the induction process and I had a meeting with the induction lead, I was horrified at how they were going to handle the allergy – it was so different from my initial enquiries. They told me that they were hands-off with support, it was entirely his own responsibility and that they wouldn't be holding a set of pens in school. They said if he forgot his AAIs/kit they would send him home as opposed to getting us to bring it into school. That felt really wrong and that they were removing themselves from any duty of care.

I was already wobbling as he was going on a public service bus with no friends at all. I could choose to fight them and get their inadequate provision corrected or see if the school that some other friends were going to had space. We hadn't previously considered it, as my son is very sporty and the school had an arts reputation, however it turns out that it is very sporty and good with allergy management!

I was able to speak in detail with the induction tutor, pastoral lead and student receptionist – who looks after the children with medical conditions and who I've built a strong relationship with. We switched and haven't looked back.'

Can I demand EpiPen training for all?

If only this were so. Being EpiPen trained is voluntary – although the Department for Health says it is 'reasonable' for all staff to be aware of the signs and symptoms of anaphylaxis, and who has been trained.[1] There is also likely to be some reliance on a child being able to self-administer.

Have this discussion with your child's school well in advance, as they should arrange training for key staff, or let you know who is trained in the event of an emergency. Your child – and pupils generally – should also be aware of who the emergency first aid lead is.

How to handle bullying

None of us want to think our child's allergies will mark them out as different, or become a target for bullying. And do take heart in the fact that teenagers today are much better informed about allergies than they were in the past.

Dan Kelly, 28, who has had nut allergies since childhood and now runs the allergy awareness blog and podcast may-contain. com, says: 'I think generally teenagers are very clued up, and with social media and all the news coverage more people are more aware about the severity of allergies.'

Of course, that's not to say the prospect of bullying should be ignored, that it never happens, or that you shouldn't be

---

1 Spare Pens in Schools: <https://www.sparepensinschools.uk/for-schools/staff-training-and-school-policies/>

prepared. A 2013 US study[2] found that almost half of parents were unaware that their children felt bullied over their food allergies. It also found that, when parents were aware, the child's quality of life improved.

The first step is to make sure lines of communication are always open – if you make it a habit to check in with your child daily, and ask open-ended questions, you will be in a better place to spot any changes in behaviour. Questions such as 'how was your day?' or 'who did you have lunch with?' are good starters.

The charity Bullying UK advises raising the topic in general conversation, at a time when you are perhaps preparing dinner, watching TV or walking the dog: ask them if they know what bullying is and what they would do if they felt they were being bullied: 'Ask what they would want to happen; this can be a great way to let them know what steps to take, such as confide in someone they trust, collect screenshots or keep a diary of incidents.'

Signs to look out for in your child include becoming withdrawn, changes in eating habits, changes in behaviour – such as becoming aggressive at home, sleeping badly, complaining of tummy aches or headaches, worrying about school, suddenly wetting the bed or suddenly doing less well at school. Of course, these don't always signify bullying, but they may arise. If they are being bullied, your child may not be ready to talk about it, so take small steps and let them know you are there. It may also help to give reassurance that you won't jump in and take action without talking to them first.

By law, all state schools must have an anti-bullying policy. This policy is decided by the school and all parents, teachers and pupils must be told what it is. The 'Keeping Children Safe in Education' guidance says schools have a duty to protect their

---

2 'Child and parental reports of bullying in a consecutive sample of children with food allergy', Shemesh et al, *Paediatrics*, 2013. See; <https://pubmed.ncbi.nlm.nih.gov/23266926/>

pupils from maltreatment; prevent impairment of children's mental and physical health or development; ensure that children grow up in circumstances consistent with the provision of safe and effective care; and take action to enable all children to have the best outcomes.

If you think there's an issue, do approach the school – but try not to storm in all guns blazing. It's very possible that your child's teacher is unaware of the situation, so give them time to assess what is going on and arrange a meeting to discuss your concerns. Having a clued-up and supportive peer group, or even just one friend, can also help. The Anaphylaxis Campaign notes: 'Encourage your child to include their friends in their allergy management. This will help if someone tries to tease them, pick on them, or bully them about their allergy.'

For more information visit <bullying.co.uk> or <bullybusters. org.uk>.

Georgia, now 24, is allergic to tree nuts, peanuts, sesame, kiwi, soya and wheat. She says: 'To any parents worried about their children starting secondary school, I would say encourage your child to learn to self-advocate before they go up. For example, when you eat out encourage them to speak to the waiter about their allergies. Speak to the school beforehand and make sure all the teachers are educated. The true friends your child makes may not understand straight away but will be willing to learn. These will become your child's 'allergy allies'. And just to add – try not to worry too much. Us allergy kids are made of pretty strong stuff.'

16

How to help your child understand and manage their allergies

As I've touched on in previous chapters, it turns out that as a general rule giving children all the information they need is a Good Idea. I'm not being facetious when I say that, because I've had my moments of wanting to protect my son from stuff that I've decided may be too serious, or too complicated. But actually I've found that being open and transparent from the outset has been best for us all.

Clinical psychologist Dr Kate Roberts says: 'In most situations children can be a bit more aware than maybe we realize, and giving them information in an age appropriate way can be a really helpful way forward. That way they can ask questions or share worries.'

A helpful way to look at it is as a gradual process of education, moving your child gently towards increasing confidence and independence. And as tempting as it is for you to take the burden and let them be carefree for as long as possible, it is good to give them small steps to take along the way. If they become slowly used to reading labels, communicating their allergies to others, recognizing symptoms and saying 'no' when they feel uncomfortable about eating something, then they will be far better equipped to handle their food allergy as teenagers and beyond, when – much as you might like – you won't always be there with a wet wipe and a packet of safe snacks. Usually.

The Anaphylaxis Campaign advises: 'Although it may be tempting for you to ask questions and read food labels on behalf of your child, remember that you are building for the future.'

We were lucky, in many ways, because my son has only ever known having allergies – having been diagnosed as a baby, he didn't have to stop eating anything he had previously enjoyed or learn a new way of life. From the moment he could bottom-shuffle across the floor we were moving food out of reach and guiding him away from anything but the food we gave him. I'd say we were also lucky in that he never made much of an effort to grab any food he wasn't allowed. I remember early birthday parties where trestle tables heaved with sandwiches, bread-sticks and cake, and unwieldy toddlers hauled themselves up to grab fistfuls of whatever they could find. For some reason, he never even tried. I had thought perhaps it was some sort of innate thing – maybe he 'knew' he had food allergies so was naturally steering clear. But other parents tell me they've had battles dragging their ravenous allergy babies away from contraband food. I suspect it may, in that case, simply be down to luck.

'Start simply – not too much complicated info. If they are asking questions then you can give a bit more. Build on that. Be led by the child. Honesty is a really good starting point because then the child will learn to trust what you are saying. Sometimes kids surprise us as to how much info they have picked up on.

Another good tip is every so often to check in and ask, "what do you know about your allergies?" to see what they say. Maybe you just do this when something new comes up, or when they have their allergy appointment, so it's a natural conversation starter. They might have completely the wrong idea!' – Dr Mary Halsey, clinical psychologist, Southampton Children's Hospital

Here are some top tips for how to help your child handle their allergies:

Toddlers

- Gentle but firm repetition of the cardinal rule 'don't touch' comes into play around food – and it helps to have an alternative to hand to show them that there is something yummy they can have; it just has to come from you.
- There's a certain amount of hygiene theatre, too – not making a fuss, but calmly cleaning down surfaces your child will eat at, so they learn not to grab food from dirty tables.
- Keep up the chat – 'we are just going to clean the table so we know there's no peanut/egg/milk here that might make you poorly'.
- The same applies to hand cleaning – a hand wash or wipe before eating and a quick reminder, 'we're just making sure your hands are clean before you eat anything'.
- When communicating your child's allergies to others, be matter-of-fact and try not to sound panicked – reiterate his or her allergies and how he or she has to eat the food you provide.
- Teach your child to only eat foods given to them by a named trusted adult – yourself, and any carers that may look after them.
- Use positive language – 'we can't have that one, but that's OK, we can have our favourite safe ice cream instead'.

Pre-schoolers

- By this stage, it's a good idea to make them familiar with their allergens: practise naming them, and make a game of pointing out the foods they are allergic to in books and supermarkets.
- Role playing is a great tool – create a doctor's set with trainer EpiPens and a mock 'allergy action plan' to demystify their medication and help them understand what it is used for.
- Similarly, use toy kitchens and toy food to talk about their allergens and how you might make safe meals and treats.
- There are some brilliant storybooks focusing on children and allergies – I mention a couple of personal favourites later in this chapter.
- Seek out TV programmes that demystify allergies for kids – the CBeebies series *Get Well Soon*, and CBBC's *Operation Ouch!*

both have handy allergy-related episodes and snippets that you can find on the BBC website or YouTube.

- Use simple language when describing an allergic reaction – 'this food will make you poorly, or give you a tummy ache/itchy rash'. If they ask questions, answer them as honestly but simply as possible.
- When buying food in a supermarket, or eating out, a gentle running narrative that explains what you are checking can be useful. ('We are just reading the label to make sure there are no nuts here ... We're just going to ask the chef if they can make something safely for you ...')
- Encourage your child to ask if they are not sure about food – and to say 'no' to anything if they don't think you have checked it's safe. This did result in my son once refusing a glass of water from an unfamiliar cup my mum offered him, but, actually, we were both quite proud of him for standing firm and it just meant we were able to have good chat about what was and wasn't OK.
- Emphasize that your child should always tell a trusted adult if they feel unwell.

Reception and Primary
- Inclusion can be a big thing by this age, so it's helpful to show your child there are alternatives even if they miss out on the odd goodie. For example, if they see a treat that they can't have, talk about how you could find a recipe to make a safe version, or emphasize all the other lovely things they can have instead.
- My son used to love going through cookbooks with me and blowing raspberries at the recipes that contained his allergens – and we would chat about what we might add or remove to make those recipes safe.
- Cooking and preparing food together can help to normalize managing allergies – using clean equipment, wiping down surfaces, checking what goes into the meal and so on.
- By the time they start school, your child should be aware that they need to wash or clean their hands before eating.
- Involve your child in preparing themselves to eat when out – perhaps they can wipe down chairs and tables themselves, then wash or clean their hands.

- Practise administering their EpiPen using a trainer pen, and talk through the signs and symptoms of an allergic reaction.
- Teach them to check they have their EpiPens every time you leave the house.
- Once they are able to read, have them help you to read food labels and menus to look for their allergens – a good tactic is to treat it like a spy mission, giving them a high five if they spot an allergen on a packet, or find a product that's safe.
- Teach them that it's perfectly OK to ask questions if they are worried – and make sure they know who the trusted adult or adults are when they are at school our without you. Who has their EpiPens? Who will be checking their food? Who should they tell if they feel poorly?

Late Primary

- By Year 6, around the age of ten, your child should be taking the first steps towards independence, as secondary school is just around the corner. By this stage, it's a good idea to have them self-carrying their medication every day, both in and out of school.
- To help them feel comfortable about self-carrying, give them the choice of bag or kit to use.
- Encourage them to have the confidence to tell other adults and parents about their allergies – for instance, when visiting friends.
- By this stage, they should begin to go into a shop alone and buy safe treats, carefully checking labels.
- Keep asking them to check labels when supermarket shopping and at home, to establish the habit.
- Help them to learn how to cook simple meals from scratch – it's a great way to embed ingredients knowledge.
- When visiting restaurants, involve them in telling staff about their allergies and helping to decide on the food they might order.
- The key thing is that these are all gentle steps, woven into everyday life.

Try to use 'we' statements rather than 'I' when you talk about managing your child's allergies – the idea behind this is to involve your child, and model behaviours they will gradually take over as they get older. Similarly, explain what you are doing out loud – 'let's get your EpiPen before we go out!'; 'let's read the label to make sure it's safe for you to eat'.

How to describe allergies to kids

We want our children to understand the seriousness of their allergies but not to scare them or make them anxious. Here are some child-friendly ways to describe allergies:

- Keep it simple – explain that some foods can make them sick, and use simple terms like 'safe food' and 'unsafe food'.
- Teach them the names of their 'unsafe foods' and what they look like by pointing them out in books, magazines and shops.
- Explain that if they are eating something and it doesn't feel right, to stop straight away and tell a grown-up.
- Use straightforward and non-scary language – for example, 'milk can make you sick, and we don't want you to be sick'.
- Explain that when someone eats something they are allergic to, their body tries to fight it – this is an allergic reaction and it can appear in different ways.
- Talk about what an allergic reaction might feel like – a tummy ache, an itchy or tickly mouth, a throat feeling a bit squeezed. Some of the descriptions in Chapter 1 may help you.

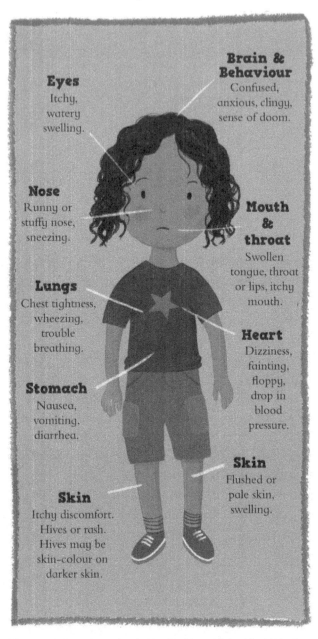

Eyes
Itchy, watery swelling.

Brain & Behaviour
Confused, anxious, clingy, sense of doom.

Nose
Runny or stuffy nose, sneezing.

Mouth & throat
Swollen tongue, throat or lips, itchy mouth.

Lungs
Chest tightness, wheezing, trouble breathing.

Heart
Dizziness, fainting, floppy, drop in blood pressure.

Stomach
Nausea, vomiting, diarrhea.

Skin
Flushed or pale skin, swelling.

Skin
Itchy discomfort. Hives or rash. Hives may be skin-colour on darker skin.

Adapted from Kath Grimshaw's book *The Cookie* published by Little Green Elephant Books <littlegreenelephantbooks.co.uk>.

How to handle the hard questions

The big question that we all fear is: 'Can I die from my allergies?' As hard as we fight to protect our kids, this realization will eventually dawn on them, and the important thing is how we respond to it. For some children, experiencing a severe reaction will be the trigger, or it may be a thoughtless chance remark by someone else. Others may take longer to get their heads around the more extreme consequences of food allergies. Equally, some may take it all in their stride.

Clinical psychologist Dr Mary Halsey says your response to the Big Question should be tailored to your child's age: 'The older the child, the more detail you can give. It's good to be honest because if a child is asking they probably already know the answer.' For older kids, she says: 'Focus on explaining that, yes, allergies can be dangerous but they can be well treated – that's the most important thing. If you are doing all of the right things, taking the right precautions and carrying your adrenaline with you, calling 999 if you have anaphylaxis, then you will be OK. That's the message to give – to focus on all of the things that they can control.'

For younger children, she advises: 'For little ones something simple like, "you are allergic to milk, which means it could make you poorly, but we've got medicine that will make you better". That might be enough, but if they are asking more then you can add a bit more info each time, so you aren't overwhelming them.' Dr Halsey adds: 'When talking, be really matter-of-fact and acknowledge yes, it is something to be careful about, but focus on what keeps them safe. We have the treatment, we have an EpiPen, we know what to do.'

For more on dealing with allergy anxieties, see Chapter 17.

Allergy books

There are a few lovely books around to help children to better understand their allergies. Here are two of my personal favourites:

The Cookie by Kath Grimshaw
You, Me and Food Allergies by Emma Amoscato

What should we carry the med kit in?

It's a good idea to choose a lightly-insulated pack where possible, as AAIs should be protected from extremes of heat or cold.

Both Yellow Cross <yellowcross.co.uk> and Medpac <medpac.co.uk> make brightly coloured (yellow and orange respectively) zip-bags, although you should know that the smaller kits will only comfortably fit two AAIs and a small bottle of antihistamine. Similar bags can be found at <allergylifestyle.com> and <theidbandco.com>. There are kid-friendly options available at <allergybuddies.com>.

When children get older, it's helpful to include them in decision-making around their kit – after all, they will have to cart it around everywhere. Some simply keep their med kits in their usual backpack. Others may prefer something smaller, in which case Medpac and others have plain, dark bumbags that can be personalized with keyrings or badges.

Some parents recommend the SPIbelt <spibelt.co.uk>, a 'low-bounce' waistband-carried bag that comes in a mix of colours and styles. There are loads of branded bumbags that teens might prefer, too, worn cross-body or around the waist. Neither of these options are insulated, but something like a FRIO Cooler case (see <allergylifestyle.com>) would fit neatly inside. Check out <diabeticsupply.co.uk> as many of their cases would double nicely as an AAI bag or kit.

If liquid antihistamines are being carried around, we've learned from bitter experience to ask the pharmacist to decant the large glass bottles into smaller plastic ones. Just remember to ask the pharmacy to stick on a prescription label, and make sure you write the expiry date on, too.

17

How to deal with anxiety

The first thing to remember is that anxiety is a perfectly natural response to stress and, as we all know, managing allergies can be hugely stressful. Previous chapters have talked a little around specific 'crunch points' like skin prick testing, and how to cope with tricky questions. But families can feel weighed down by a general sense of anxiety around daily life too.

For parents, it's the unrelenting weight of constant vigilance and uncertainty. Children may start to feel anxious in the wake of a reaction, or perhaps they are scared to take those first steps to independence – telling others about their allergies or ordering food when eating out. There is also a fine line between caution and fear, and it's one that we all find difficult to tread sometimes. It's really important to know that you are not alone.

My experience – I have no idea if true for all – is that it tends to come in waves. I'll have bursts of organizing energy and campaigning zeal, trying new products, ringing manufacturers, eating at a new restaurant and coming away excited by the possibilities. At other times, it weighs heavy: I'll see my youngest daughter – allergy free – skipping off to enjoy a Chinese meal for her friend's birthday and it will hit me that my son just can't do those things in the same way, with such carefree abandon. Or I'll give my daughter a silly sloppy kiss on the lips and it will strike me that I've never – not ever – done that unthinkingly with my son, because of the all-pervasive fear that something I've eaten might cause a reaction.

Perhaps life, or work, or something else, is causing background agitation and the idea of trying something as simple as a new ice cream, or going through the 'allergy rigmarole' in a restaurant, just seems like a hurdle too far. And then I start to think about upcoming events – a school trip, a party, secondary school – and the anxiety fizzes up.

In this chapter I try to cover a little about some of the common anxiety triggers (both for children and parents), what support you can access, and some handy resources for managing those generalized feelings of worry when they arise.

The state of things

Psychological services for allergy aren't where they should be, but there is a move to improve them. A 2019 study[1] led by Dr Rebecca Knibb, reader in psychology at Aston University, identified the 'unmet need' in psychological services for families and parents of children with food allergy. The study notes: 'Management of food allergy involves constant vigilance [and] research has demonstrated that this burden, along with the unpredictable nature of allergic reactions, has an impact on quality of life and mental health, including stress, worry, anxiety and depression.' It pinpoints the 'paucity of psychological services to support families coping with this condition'.

Meanwhile, clinical psychologist Dr Kate Roberts' 2021 study[2] found 81 per cent of parents of children with food allergy reported 'clinically significant worry' and more than 42 per cent met the clinical cut-off for Post-Traumatic Stress Syndrome (PTSS). Dr Roberts' paper also suggested there is a link between intolerance of uncertainty and anxiety when it comes to food allergy – in other words, finding the

1 'Psychological services for food allergy: the unmet need for patients and families in the United Kingdom', Knibb et al, *Clinical & Experimental Allergy, 2019*. See: <https://onlinelibrary.wiley.com/doi/abs/10.1111/cea.13488>

2 'Parental Anxiety and Posttraumatic Stress Symptoms (PTSS) in Paediatric Food Allergy', Roberts et al, *Journal of Paediatric Psychology*, 2021. See: <https://pubmed.ncbi.nlm.nih.gov/33704484/>

uncertainty of the condition hard to tolerate. 'Obviously, caring for a child with food allergy involves a lot of uncertainty, for example around attending social events where food will be served,' she says. Uncertainty is also built into diagnosis because there is no test to predict the severity of any potential future reaction. She says the evidence suggests that 'talking therapies' such as Cognitive Behavioural Therapy (CBT) can help to break down negative thought patterns and ease anxiety.

There are currently only two paediatric allergy clinics in the UK with funding for dedicated clinical psychology services – Southampton General Hospital and the Evelina London Children's Hospital. Both of these show that early psychological intervention can help – such as the 'stepped care' at the Evelina, which runs workshops on cognitive behavioural therapy techniques for parents and children, as well as key areas such as 'improving communication with schools' or 'preparing for skin prick tests'.

Unfortunately, these services are not widely available but the moral of the story for now is: the burden of coping with food allergy is considerable. You are far from alone if you're feeling anxious, and you should always tell your allergy specialist or GP if these feelings are becoming a barrier to your quality of life. Dr Mary Halsey, clinical psychologist in the paediatric allergy service at Southampton hospital, says: 'There are various research projects ongoing and the hope is that we can convince more services to see the need for specialized psychological support for allergy. It will need time, but I think it will grow.'

How do I get help?

'There's a justification for seeking help if you get to the point where you are thinking, "this is affecting how we are living, or worrying is taking up a lot of my time, or it's affecting my sleep or sapping my mental energy",' says Dr Kate Roberts. 'For instance, even if you are managing to take your child to normal events, when you are there you find your heart is always racing, you're feeling a bit shaky, you're not enjoying the experience. Of course, we all have moments of anxiety but this is a level where it's having a persistent negative impact for you in some way.'

First ask your allergy clinic if they have any psychological support services – some may be running small-scale studies or trials that you can take part in as anxiety and food allergy is an emerging area of research. If this is not available, go to your GP and tell them you are really struggling with anxiety linked to your child's allergies. They should be able to signpost to appropriate services in your local area.

In England you can also self-refer to NHS psychological therapies (IAPT) services for free, including CBT and counselling. See <https://www.nhs.uk/service-search/find-a-psychological -therapies-service/> for more information.

In Scotland, visit the Scottish Association for Mental Health website at <samh.org.uk> to find support, or see <https:// www.nhsinform.scot/illnesses-and-conditions/mental-health/ anxiety>. In Wales and Northern Ireland, referral is via your GP as there are currently no self-referral services.

If your child is the one feeling anxious, talk to your allergy team, or ask your GP to signpost you to services, such CAMHS (Child and Adolescent Mental Health Services) or local free counselling. Some schools have counsellors available, too. Clinical psychologist Dr Mary Halsey reassures: 'Even if you can't access specialist allergy counselling and they may not be a trained allergy psychologist, these services will have very good training to help children with anxiety. Sometimes they might even liaise with the specialist allergy nurses in your clinic, which can help. So do ask for help if you think you need it.'

Find out the cause

Very often, an anxiety around one thing will stem from something else. For example, it is quite common for children displaying fear around eating new foods, or eating out, to actually have an underlying phobia about their adrenaline injector.

Dr Mary Halsey says: 'We do find EpiPen phobia comes up quite a lot in clinic. It might be a fear of needles and a fear of the unknown. Tackling the anxiety is about getting to the crux of what it's about. I've seen children who, when they have been able to overcome that EpiPen phobia, have started to eat more of a varied diet and try new things again – safely, of course.'

If you can tease out the crux of a worry, you might find it's fairly easily resolved – very often, a fear around EpiPens turns out to be a worry that the needle is the same length as the whole pen. Dr Halsey advises asking a child to draw what they think an EpiPen looks like inside, and finding patient information on the manufacturers' websites to show the reality. Other children are convinced it will be very painful, which, as Dr Halsey points out too, 'is really not what people say' (see Chapter 2 for more about people's experiences of using an AAI).

Recognizing the signs

Sometimes your child's anxiety is crystal clear, and you can start to get to grips with what is worrying them quite quickly. At other times, they may harbour worries secretly. So what signs should you watch out for to see if anxiety is starting to creep into their thoughts?

Signs of worry around food may include not eating their lunch at school, or losing weight. They may start to avoid activities, such as having tea at their friend's house, or show reluctance at school trips or parties. It's obviously hard to know whether these things are sparked by allergy anxiety – and it takes a little detective work.

Dr Halsey says: 'Look out for subtle signs of avoidance or saying they aren't interested in going out or socializing. It may well be that they are, but they are scared. Other signs may be they are a bit withdrawn or not seeming like themselves. Children that don't really want to talk about their allergies can be a bit of a sign because – why not? Are they avoiding talking about allergies?'

How to talk about your child's worries

The best approach is the least pressured one. Weaving questions into conversation, rather than demanding a sit-down chat, can herald the best results.

Dr Halsey says: 'Coax worries out – use anything that's less intense like going on a dog walk or, with younger children, when they are in the bath. Use opportunities where you are doing something else at the same time. You could use your visit to the allergy clinic or to the chemist to get their new EpiPens as a natural opportunity to say, "how are you feeling about your allergies at the moment?" '

Another tactic recommended by clinical psychologists is 'externalizing' anxiety. Dr Halsey explains: 'If your child has a worry, ask them, "what is the worry saying to you?" It takes the worry outside of the child – talking about 'the worry' rather than 'your worry'. So you might say, "when you're feeling nervous, what does the worry say to you? What happens when that worry is there? What does it make you want to do or not do? What does it make you want to avoid?" '

She also recommends reassurance that the worry is perfectly understandable – but not necessarily 'true'. 'You might start a conversation around the worrying being really normal and natural: when you have allergies you have to be wary and keep an eye out, and sometimes that tips over into worry and that's understandable,' she says. 'We'd say, the worry is the body's alarm system that tells you if something might be dangerous, but in a lot of situations that alarm is a false alarm – like a smoke detector that goes off when you make toast. It normalizes and validates the child's worries.'

Another tactic – when your child is in upper primary and old enough to realize worries aren't true – is to ask your child to write down their worry on one side of a piece of paper. For example, if they are scared to try a new cereal bar, they might write 'I'm scared it will have peanuts in it'. On the other side, ask them to write down the truth – which they have to come up with. So, it might be, 'I've checked the label and there are no peanuts in the cereal bar.' Dr Halsey explains: 'It's about differentiating the worry from the truth.'

Use the gradual exposure ladder

This is a tried and tested cognitive behavioural therapy (CBT) tool for managing anxiety, and can be adopted for a wide range of different scenarios. The idea is that you create a 'ladder' of small steps towards an agreed goal. For example, if your child has an EpiPen phobia, you would work together to write down all the things they could do to practice with their pen – working up from least scary, to most scary. Each of these is a step up on the ladder.

Impressively, at Southampton Children's Hospital, children who are EpiPen-phobic and have worked up the ladder are invited into the day ward and, under supervision, helped to inject themselves with their AAI. Obviously this isn't a 'try this at home' scenario and very few allergy clinics have the resources to offer this, so something less dramatic might be at the top of your ladder – such as injecting an expired EpiPen into an orange, which, for some children, can feel frighteningly real.

Steps should be small and manageable, beginning with something as simple as holding a practice EpiPen, or looking at a picture of an EpiPen, moving through things such as using the trainer pen on a soft toy, or watching a parent do it. Dr Halsey says: 'It's a nice way for the child to gain confidence in a way that's manageable for them. It's like desensitizing, really, and a good technique for anxiety generally.'

Top tips include:

- Go at your child's pace, albeit with gentle encouragement, and help to move up the ladder.
- Do it a few times before trying to move to the next rung.
- If your child gets 'stuck', break the next rung down into tinier steps – if they can't inject an orange, what about doing it with a trainer pen, then watching a video of someone else doing it, and so on.
- Make sure your child is the one to create the ladder, to give them a sense of control.
- Remember their steps may surprise you, in terms of what they find more or less scary, but it has to be their own experience.
- Keep a copy of the 'ladder' somewhere they are happy with – on a wall, inside a cupboard door, or in a drawer.
- Agree between you when you will move on to the next step.
- Try not to make it pressurized, and don't feel you need to do this every day.

This gradual exposure technique can be used for all ages and scenarios: for example, if they are nervous about eating out, or trying something new, you might begin by trying a different loaf of bread from a trusted brand, then a different (safe) brand, and so on to their goal. 'Anxiety is built around avoidance, so you want to help your children not to avoid these situations,' adds Dr Halsey.

If they are scared of eating out, you might start by visiting the restaurant and looking at the menu from outside, then popping in briefly and asking to see the allergy menu, moving up to having a drink but no meal, until your child feels gradually more comfortable and you can order a small dish. 'Anxiety can feel really overwhelming – there will be lots of worries and beliefs and we want our children to learn these things aren't inherently dangerous. We need them to experience that that worry didn't come true. "You had that different type of biscuit and the worry didn't come true". It's really powerful,' adds Dr Halsey.

Coping after anaphylaxis

If a child has been through a frightening event, such as a serious reaction, you might notice they:

- become upset easily;
- are a bit tearful;
- don't sleep well;
- lose their appetite.

Dr Halsey says: 'These would be typical and perfectly normal reactions for a time, but if that persists say beyond a couple of months, or if the anxiety is overwhelming, then maybe they might need some help with it.' The advice, she says, is to give them space to talk about what happened but without pressure. Let them know that if they are upset, it's OK. Perhaps they might be comfortable speaking to someone else – a close family member or friend, for example. 'Help them come up with a narrative with a beginning, middle and end for what happened – so, we were in that café, I had that cake and it had peanut in, I felt ill and these were my symptoms, and we gave the EpiPen and called an ambulance ... and now I am OK and I am at home again. With traumatic events memories can get stuck and it can feel like it's still happening. This helps them know it's now OK.

It places them back in the here and now – they are safe and, if it happens again, they are going to be safe because you know what to do.'

Sometimes these worries can linger and present themselves further down the line in issues such as anxiety about eating, or going out – in which case the 'graded exposure' technique (above) is a helpful tool.

Of course, coping after a serious reaction can be traumatic for parents or carers too. A 2021 study[3] led by clinical psychologist Dr Kate Roberts found that, for 60 per cent of parents of children with food allergy, witnessing their child's anaphylactic reaction was the most stressful event they had ever faced. While some may feel more confident knowing they managed to handle the reaction well, others may end up feeling more anxious and risk-averse.

Dr Roberts says: 'With any traumatic incident it's quite normal for the first week or two afterwards to need to process what has happened – you may have nightmares, or vivid memories, or increased anxiety. But if either you are highly distressed or if things are persisting then do see your GP.'

The same 'normalization strategies' you might try with your child could help you, too – reminding yourself that what you have been through was indeed frightening and a threat, but that, in the here and now, you and your child are safe. Calming breathing exercises can also help when you feel your anxiety spiralling, and particularly if you build them into your normal routine.

The NHS website has self-help strategies for improving mental health at <https://www.nhs.uk/mental-health/self-help/guides-tools-and-activities/>. They advise the following breathing

---

3 'Parental Anxiety and Posttraumatic Stress Symptoms in Paediatric Food Allergy', Roberts et al, *Journal of Paediatric Psychology*, 2021. See: <https://academic.oup.com/jpepsy/advance-article-abstract/doi/10.1093/jpepsy/jsab012/6163077?redirectedFrom=fulltext>

technique, which you can do standing, sitting in a supportive chair or lying down:

- Make yourself comfortable and loosen restrictive clothes.
- If lying down, place your arms a little bit away from your sides, palms up. Let your legs be straight or bend your knees so your feet are flat on the floor.
- If sitting, place your arms on the chair arms or loosely in your lap.
- If sitting or standing, place feet flat on the ground and roughly hip-width apart.
- Let your breath flow as deep into your belly as is comfortable, without forcing it.
- Try to breathe in through your nose and out through your mouth.
- Breathe in gently and regularly – you might like to count steadily from one to five.
- Without pause or holding your breath let it flow out gently, counting again from one to five if this helps.
- Continue for three to five minutes.

Other tips include muscle relaxation – tensing, then releasing, muscles in your body – and gentle exercise, such as going for a walk, swim, cycle, doing yoga, or even active distractions such as gardening or doing housework.

Keep calm to teach calm

As we all know, kids pick up on adults' worries and emotions, so the first step towards helping your child manage their fears is to manage your own.

'It's really important that the adult feels confident,' says Dr Halsey. 'I would always encourage adults just to seek out allergy info to make sure they are comfortable with what is OK and what is not. And if anxiety is getting the better of them, they should absolutely seek support in their own right.'

Modelling calm behaviour is also key – but hard! If you find yourself in a situation – a kids' party, say, where there is lots of food flying about – try not to panic (easier said than done). Dr Halsey says: 'If you're calm and matter-of-fact then that's what the child learns. It's so hard to do when you aren't feeling it, but in a situation like that, rather than saying, "oh no let's not go over there" you might say "right, let's have a look first and see if it's OK." If you feel your anxiety rising, find a way if possible to step back – nip to the loo, for instance, and think, "what is it I'm worried about? Do I need to be extra cautious? What can I do here?" It's also about being realistic – there are situations that are a bit uncertain so it's OK to let a little bit of worry show. "Mummy just needs to work out what we can do here, then we'll be OK." Try to model that matter-of-fact approach.'

Another good tip is to recruit another adult to accompany you to stressful situations – ideally one who is less anxious than you (although blasé isn't helpful, either!). You could take your partner, or ask a fellow parent or friend at the party to help you keep an eye out. And if the activity or event is just too much, and you feel it isn't safe, don't be scared to step away. Just be calm in how you explain this to your child, so they don't start to fear or avoid future similar occasions. If they are very young, you can pretend there's another reason to leave; if they are older you might explain that it wasn't an appropriate situation to be in – they were decorating biscuits with peanuts, say, or having a food fight – but that it is exceptional, and things like this don't often happen.

I'm too scared to give my child anything new to eat

We have all felt it, to one degree or another. Find me the allergy parent who hasn't at least once fished packaging out of the bin just to double (triple) check a new item of food is definitely, absolutely, completely safe.

It's important that we all double-check labels, of course. There have been times when the rush to throw food in the supermarket trolley has ended up with us bringing home something we later realize, despite looking, has egg in, or a sesame warning. But it's when the vigilance tips into fear that we need to take steps to manage our feelings.

'I'm just so scared to let my daughter try anything new, even if I've checked the label, know it's a trustworthy brand, and have asked other allergy parents too. I know I need to let her try things, but so often I just don't know how to do it. I am so scared to let her touch anything.'

'Oh my god I often root around in the bin to check ingredients, even after I know I've already checked and it's fine ...'

'I literally can't stop looking at labels and rechecking a million times.'

'Sometimes I'm on the train to work and I worry about what I have put in his lunchbox, even though it's stuff he has eaten before.'

'I'll check to see if my son is still alive if I've given him a new food in the early evening and he's gone to bed – even though there's been no sign of a reaction and no reason to fear one.'

'If we are eating somewhere new I'm on hyper-alert, scrutinizing his face for the tiniest hint of a red mark, or sitting up like a meercat if he clears his throat. Honestly, it's completely exhausting.'

Dr Mary Halsey says: 'This is a very common anxiety that we see a lot, in both children and parents. The problem with over-checking or constantly asking for reassurance is that the more we do it the more of a habit it becomes. For example, if we aren't sure then it is completely appropriate to check twice, as any allergy team would recommend. But if we are checking packets multiple times due to worry, then we come to rely on doing just that. There is a sense of relief that comes from checking multiple times and this can serve to reinforce the checking. Therefore we become reliant on over-checking.'

So how to manage it? Dr Halsey advises setting some clear rules (brace yourselves – it won't be easy but it's worth it): 'For example, if the food is safe – it doesn't contain any allergens – then we allow ourselves to check twice. Then, any urge to check or anxiety that we feel, we must try to tolerate this and "sit with" the anxiety. This is of course difficult, but it is the only way to break the cycle.' She adds: 'Once the parent sees that the child is OK, then this will reinforce the fact that they didn't need to check again. Parents could start with "easier" food items without the child even knowing that this is what the parent is doing. You could also ask for support from their co-parent or a relative/friend, to help you to not check a third time. And if this isn't manageable then you can seek help from your allergy team or GP. There are services out there that can help.'

Reassurance seeking

This takes us on to another common habit in anxious children – constant seeking of reassurance. Your instinct may well be to give that reassurance, to soothe them and show that you are looking out for them. But Dr Halsey warns this may be counter-productive. 'If a child seeks reassurance multiple times then it's better to use that as an opportunity to say "I can see you're worried, what is the worry saying to you? What can you say back to the worry/what is the truth of the situation?" You're getting them to manage their own worry, which is more helpful than giving them yet more reassurance, which they may come to rely on. This helps with their confidence too as they can manage the worry themselves and therefore can do this if the parent, or adult, isn't around.'

Handy resources for managing anxiety

Allergy charities

Both the Anaphylaxis Campaign and Allergy UK have great advice on their websites for dealing with anxiety around allergies. See <anaphylaxis.org.uk> and <allergyuk.org>.

Evelina London

The Evelina Children's Hospital in London has an impressive range of patients' leaflets online, on topics including managing anxiety. Head to <www.evelinalondon.nhs.uk/our-services/hospital/allergy-service/patient-leaflets.aspx>.

Websites

YoungMinds – this UK charity has guidance for children and young people managing their mental health. Visit <youngminds.org.uk/>.

Anxiety Canada – ignore the Canada bit, this is a brilliant website recommended by clinical psychologists, with practical strategies and tools to manage anxiety in children, including a free online plan and downloadable PDFs. See <anxietycanada.com>.

NHS – the NHS website has info-packed sections dedicated to mental health, with self-help ideas and general advice. Head to <nhs.uk/mental-health>.

Apps

Headspace – a very helpful and popular mindfulness app. Check out the website at <headspace.com> for some anxiety advice too.

Smiling Mind – a daily mindfulness and meditation guide with free programmes for children as well as adults.

MindShift – an app designed to help teens and young adults cope with anxiety, from the team behind Anxiety Canada.

Books

Ruby's Worry by Tom Percival

The Worrysaurus by Rachel Bright

No Worries: Mindful Kids activity book by Dr Sharie Coombes and Katie Abey

The Huge Bag of Worries by Virginia Ironside

Happy: A Children's Book of Mindfulness by Nicola Edwards and Katie Hickey

The Worrying Worries by Rachel Rooney

My Monster and Me by Nadiya Hussein

The HappySelf Journal (see <happyselfjournal.com>)

Helping Your Child With Worry and Anxiety by Ann Cox

Worry Monsters and more

Some families find a physical repository for their child's worries can be a huge help. You may want to make or buy a worry monster – cuddly soft monsters with big mouths. Children write their worries on a piece of paper and feed them to their monster. The Evelina London has even introduced one to its allergy clinic.

Worry dolls are also a nice idea – again, you can buy them, or children can make their own. The idea is that your child tells their worries to the dolls before bed, pops them under their pillow and they will absorb those worries.

A worry box is another tactic – children write their worries down, read them aloud, and put them inside. Or you could encourage your child to visualize their worry being put into a box and on a boat, and for that boat to sail away into the far distance.

Tips for managing general anxiety in young children

The Evelina London has some handy online tips at <www. evelinalondon.nhs.uk/resources/patient-information/managing-your-anxiety.pdf>. These include:

- Create a routine – have visual timetables or lists so your child knows what is happening day-to-day and can feel more in control.
- Distraction – if your child is feeling anxious, try distracting them with games such as 'I spy', counting or naming things they see, reading, watching TV, colouring or listening to music.
- Exercise – young children can try star jumps, hide and seek, skipping; or for older children going for a bike ride, swimming or climbing can help.
- Bumblebee breathing – place the tips of your index fingers in your ears and close your eyes. Slowly breathe in through your nose and hum quietly as you breathe out.

Sara Smillie's son Calum was diagnosed with allergies at seven, following an anaphylactic reaction to peanuts. She talks about the anxieties he faced as a young child and how she helped him to overcome them:

'When he was about eight, Calum started having nightmares that he was being force fed peanuts. At the same time, he started asking, "can my allergies kill me?" As soon as he brought it up, we asked his allergist for a therapy referral, which seemed to help him after just one visit. We also spoke to him and reassured him by putting all the following into place: firstly, we let him know that we had none of his allergens in the house and none of us ate his allergens, which was reassuring for him. I do appreciate that not everyone can do that. I

think it's about putting rules and systems into action and letting every child know from an early age that they are there to protect them.

I made an information sheet with Calum's help and listed all the signs and symptoms of a reaction, Calum's date of birth, his allergies, our phone numbers as well as an action plan, and I showed everyone from babysitters to family – everyone who was coming to our house was told about his allergies. To this day it is still taped to the inside of our cupboard door. We also asked everyone to wash their hands on entering our house. All these little things that I introduced added up to reassure Calum that he was safe. We always spoke about these rules with Calum and his brother and we still follow them to this day. He's now 25!'

18

Holidays and travel

I don't *think* holidays figure in the list of top ten most stressful life events – you know the ones: divorce, bereavement, moving house, losing your job ... But I bet you pretty much every allergy family would add a number 11 in a heartbeat: 'travel'.

The idea of holidaying away from home – abroad, specifically – can be the straw that breaks the allergy camel's back. It's not uncommon to discover that parents of children with allergies have made a conscious decision not to take the risk. And it's not simply that they think it's inherently unsafe to travel overseas; many will concede that it is probably perfectly possible. But it's the overwhelming burden of preparation and worry that comes with it.

The logistics of travel – planes, trains, ferries – language barriers, unknown supermarkets, mysterious healthcare systems, trusting in someone new to cater every meal. Sometimes it all just feels too much. If you spend every meal out when on home turf staring at your child in case a hive pops up, imagine the stress of doing that same thing every day for two weeks? That's not a holiday.

But.

I'm not here to tell you that it comes without prep, or stress, or even the occasional hitch. With careful planning in place, though, you can do it.

Taking your first trip

Where should you start? If you're nervous, there are a few obvious choices that can make a first trip away feel more manageable. Go easy on yourself to begin with – you can go bigger and bolder as you gain more confidence.

Choose self-catering

Pick a property with a good kitchen. Make sure that what looks like an oven is actually an oven: we once made the rudimentary error of booking an apartment with what turned out to be only a posh-looking microwave and a kettle, which made cooking pizzas a bit of a challenge ...

Find a big name supermarket

Go for a location close to a large-ish supermarket. Do a bit of research beforehand to find the major retailers and see if they label allergens well. Generally, you'll find big name food shops have clear labelling.

Start small

Don't pressurize yourself into making a round-the-world trip from the off. Consider a destination that doesn't feel like a challenge to get to for your first trip abroad. A long journey can be fraught and tiring at the best of times.

Look for the familiar

Pick somewhere you know – choose a location you've visited before and feel comfortable with. Maybe you speak the language (or bits of it) or can navigate your way around fairly easily.

Stick to the beaten track

Opt for somewhere that isn't far off the beaten track – for a first step, you'll feel less anxious if you are close to a large conurbation where there are big shops, healthcare facilities, and so on.

Do your research

Ask other allergy families for recommendations – there are several Facebook forums set up for families managing allergies, and good communities on Instagram and Twitter. If you can, go to one of the support groups run by your allergy clinic or the Anaphylaxis Campaign and ask for tips there. If family members or friends are visiting a hotel or resort, give them a list of questions to ask so you can suss out whether they might be allergy friendly or not. Check Tripadvisor by popping 'allergies' or 'allergy friendly' into the search bar.

Checklist of things to remember

There are a few basics to remember when you travel. Here's a handy list to get you started:

- Make sure medication is in date and consider taking extra supplies as back-up.
- Find out where the nearest emergency department is, and what the number for emergency services is.
- Check whether your insurance covers you for allergies – you'll need to declare the condition, and make sure you're protected for emergency treatment, ambulance transfers, hospital admissions and replacement of medication. The Anaphylaxis Campaign has a helpful online database of insurance firms and their allergy cover at <anaphylaxis. org.uk>.
- Consider using a translation card. These detail your child's allergies and requirements when you're eating out, or need medical assistance, and are available in a wide range of languages. Visit <allergyaction.org> or Allergy UK at <allergyuk.org/get-help/translation-cards>.
- Check food labelling laws in the country you are visiting. They are the same across the EU, and currently the same as in the UK, but Australia, New Zealand, the US and other countries have their own regulations. You can check on the

University of Nebraska-Lincoln's Food Allergy Research and Resource Program website at <farrp.unl.edu/IRChart>.

Our story

I have family in Italy so we were lucky in that we could start gently – in a city we knew well, with a language I can speak, and people we knew close by. Even so, I found myself surprised by how allergy friendly it actually was.

Visiting a country without allergies, and visiting one with allergies, are very different experiences. Don't assume it's impossible based on what you've eaten before. By this I mean that you might think, 'Gah! Italy! Ice creams, pizzas, milk, hazelnuts everywhere ...' But if you've travelled without allergies you will never have had an eye out for what is available for those with special dietary needs.

When we did start looking, we found an amazing selection of 'free from' foods in supermarkets, excellent product labelling from some of the big name retailers and lots of people incredibly willing to help. In fact, we've found food in the shops there that I've yet to find back home – sesame-free grissini, for instance, and milk-, egg- and nut-free tarts and croissants. When we go, we stock up and cart a stash back home with us to keep us going until the next trip.

We even found the major manufacturers had brilliant consumer helplines – dare I say better than in the UK. On one trip, we came across what looked like a safe ice lolly, and rang the number on the packaging – it was Algida, the Italian version of Wall's. Within minutes I had spoken to someone clear and knowledgeable, and that lolly was swiftly in the fist of my then very happy four-year-old.

What to pack

I recall with misty eyes the days when packing for holidays meant three bikinis, a couple of sundresses, suncream and a lipstick. These days clothes and toiletries have given way to the contents of a supermarket trolley.

Over the years I've refined our food packing to the things we usually end up needing. When I say 'refined', I don't mean Marie Kondo-minimized – I mean it used to be the contents of *two* supermarket trolleys. As one fellow allergy parent puts it, 'It takes the best part of a week and a whole suitcase of food when we travel!'

What you pack will depend on where you're going and your allergies, but here are a few suggestions that we've found helpful when holidaying abroad. (Note: if you're carting food to foreign climes, do check what the import restrictions are at your destination – some countries may have limits on the transportation of meat, fruit and vegetables, for example.)

Food

- **Breads and crackers** – Whether you're gluten free or sesame free, it can be tricky finding safe baked goods. I pack savoury biscuits, breadsticks and breads that don't perish too quickly. Pittas and wraps are good and pack flat, too. Crumpets and safe croissants can be useful. If we're travelling to Italy, I'll add a ciabatta or similar so we can 'match' fresh breads when eating out.
- **Chocolate and treats** – These can also be hard to find, so I always pack biscuits, favourite chocolate bars and non-perishable cakes from companies such as Lazy Day Foods. So handy to have back-up when you just can't track down a safe ice cream, or you're eating out somewhere where the desserts aren't allergy friendly. Shelf-stable jelly or custard pots are useful.
- **Pizza bases** – It seems ridiculous taking pizzas to Italy, but we do always pack a couple in case we want to eat out as a family but can't find somewhere safe. Generally speaking, restaurants have been hugely helpful and understanding when we've asked if they mind us bringing our son's food. Usually, I'll cook his in the apartment before we head out, and pack it in a foil container, but some places have kindly offered to heat up our food. I only say 'yes' if they clearly understand the need to avoid cross contamination.

- **Avocado** – If you can take fruit or veg, I find a couple of unripe avocados in the suitcase a really handy back-up in emergencies. It's virtually a meal in itself with a few crackers in the event you find nothing else.
- **Dried fruit and porridge sachets, mini packs of cereal** – Breakfast in an instant.
- **Milk and cheese alternatives** – Unless you know your destination is well set for dairy free options, packing some of your favourites is always a good idea.
- **Cereal bars and kid snacks**
- **Flour** – If you need a specialist flour, pack a small one just in case.
- **Ready to bake** – Sometimes I take the dry mix to bake fresh scones or a cake – I measure out the sugar, flour, baking powder and so on, seal it in a plastic freezer bag and pop it into a Tupperware in the suitcase. Especially handy if travelling on family birthdays. Pack cupcake cases too if needed.
- **Safe staple** – A safe packet of pasta, cous cous or rice is a good fallback in case you struggle to find something suitable.
- **First meal** – Sometimes it takes a day or two to suss out the local shops, so having a meal ready to go for the first night is a good plan. A quick pasta and packet sauce, or an ambient (non-chilled) ready meal can do the trick.
- **Dessert toppings** – You may find a safe pudding or ice cream when you're away, but if a sibling's dessert comes piled high with chocolate curls and glacé cherries, you'll want a quick fix to appease your child with allergies. I pack mini marshmallows and safe sprinkles just in case.

Equipment

- **Foil and foil trays** – If you're going to be carting food about, don't forget to pack a few pots and wrappers for storing cooked meals or sandwiches and snacks.

- **A wooden spoon and a frying pan** – Two more things I stuff in the suitcase. I never use other people's wooden utensils, because they can soak up allergens and oils, and I sometimes have a frying pan to hand in case I'm not happy with the cookware.

- **Cheese grater** – Another item that's often missing in apartments but that proves handy. I have a mini one especially for travel.

- **Foldable colander** – If we are staying in a hotel and I want to cater some meals myself, then having a portable colander is helpful for washing fresh fruit, salad and veg, or cooking up a quick pasta dish.

- **Chopping board** – As one fellow allergy parent notes, 'there's nothing worse than wondering what it's been used for before.' You can buy handy roll-up ones for easy packing.

- **A sharp knife and portable cutlery** – This is a good call when you're staying in a hotel and realize you only have a toothbrush to cut cheese and butter bread with.

- **Remoska** – What's that, I hear you cry? An amazing thing! We stumbled across these in Lakeland. It's not cheap, but if you travel a lot and don't always have access to self-catering, then it repays the cost. It's essentially a plug-in electric saucepan on a base that cooks food like an oven. You need a power source to use it, but it's great for cooking up a stew, or heating through a ready meal, when you don't have self-catering options. We haven't been too adventurous yet but apparently they can cook baked potatoes, roast chicken, toasted sandwiches, heat up a pre-packed mini pizza and even prepare a fry-up. (Top tip: If you buy one, also buy the rack to go in it.)

Don't forget, adrenaline pens don't like extremes of heat or cold – so don't leave them in direct sunlight, or store them in a fridge. You can buy insulated med packs to keep them at an even temperature (see Chapter 16 for details).

Hotel checklist

Very much like arranging to eat in a restaurant, staying in a hotel or resort requires some prep. Your first step, of course, is research – ask for recommendations, scour allergy-friendly travel blogs, look at online reviews. But once you've tracked down somewhere promising here's a quick rundown of key things to ask:

• Can they cater for allergies at every meal?
• How do they handle buffets? Can they provide freshly cooked alternatives served separately?
• Do they have a catering manager who oversees all dining? If so, ask to have a conversation with that person directly, and introduce yourself on arrival.
• Can they check every ingredient for 'may contain' warnings (if you avoid them) and prepare food free from cross contamination?
• Are there any foods they may struggle to source – bread, for instance, or desserts? Can they buy anything in for you before you arrive, or are they happy for you to bring your own alternatives (for instance, we often travel with safe bread and cereals).
• Can they store any food you bring in their fridge or freezer, if needed?
• Who will be the named person responsible for overseeing your food during your stay? Will they be on-site all the time?

- Should you pre-order your child's meals?
- Can they check with manufacturers whether the ice creams on-site are safe?
- Do they have medical facilities or a hospital nearby?

Also:

- **Ask for a hot plate** – If you're staying at a hotel or resort and feel you need the option to self-cater a meal or two, ask if they will provide a hot plate in your room. We have had this on several occasions, and it's been really helpful for cooking up a quick pasta dish or a hot wrap.
- **Empty the mini bar** – Ask in advance if they can empty the mini bar of any nuts or fresh milk. Handily an empty mini bar also gives room for you to store your own food stash. We take deli meats, olives and other bits for my son.
- **Watch out for free snacks** – You might find your hotel delivers foodie treats to your room every so often as a complimentary gift. Have a chat with hotel management before your stay, or on check-in, to make sure you don't come back from a day at the beach to find peanut brittle on your pillow.

Websites and resources for travelling with allergies

Websites and blogs spring up all the time, and a quick Google search can throw up lots of options. Here are a few tried and tested sites that may help your research:

International allergy organizations

Check the allergy charities or organizations in the country you are visiting. The Anaphylaxis Campaign has a helpful list in the 'travel' section of their website. These organizations may be able to offer additional support and advice.

Facebook

There are several Facebook groups dedicated to eating out and travelling with allergies. They tend to be US-based as a whole, but can include some helpful tips and starting points when researching new places to go. Try the Allergy Travels group and also Peanut and Nut Allergy Travel Tips.

Finding milk-free options

Although its target audience is vegan, the website <happycow. net> can pick out food stores that sell vegan products in hundreds of locations across the globe – useful if you are struggling to find a milk alternative or similar. Bear in mind, though, that vegan does not mean allergy friendly, so never automatically assume that the dining out recommendations are safe.

US travel

The website <allergyeats.com> has reviews and guides to allergy-friendly places to eat across the USA. On Facebook, the US-based Dining Out with Food Allergies group can be very helpful. If Disney is in your sights, the <allergyfreemouse.com> blog and review sight is a good starting point. And <nutfreenewyork.com> is one person's handy guide to nut allergy-friendly places to eat.

Allergy bloggers

There are a few long-standing allergy bloggers out there. For some starter travel tips try Miss Allergic Reactor <missallergicreactor.com>, Gluten Free Cuppa Tea <glutenfreecuppatea.co.uk> and <thezestfull.com>.

The UK children's charity Over the Wall runs holiday camps for children aged 8 to 17 with serious medical conditions. These include residential trips for those with severe or multiple allergies – where the children have fully trained staff on hand to manage their needs, and an impressive menu of allergy-safe food. See <otw.org.uk> for details.

Flying safely

If you're already a nervous flyer, as I am, adding the burden of allergies on top can be extremely stressful. But the one thing you need to know is that it is perfectly possible to fly safely with allergies, and there are just a few steps you can take to ease your mind and mitigate any potential risks.

Nuts on planes

One of the biggest worries for families, which comes up time and again, is that of in-flight snacks and the potential for an aircraft full of people to be chomping – for example – on tree nuts or peanuts 35,000ft up in the air. This is an issue that often divides – those who insist nuts on planes pose little risk, those who insist nuts on planes are automatically deadly, and those who sit somewhere in between.

First – the science. Studies have shown that shelling peanuts is highly unlikely to result in peanut particles becoming and remaining airborne. There is also currently no evidence to suggest that peanut dust circulates and causes reactions. Many experts believe that reactions are far more likely to come from surface contamination – so trays or tables being contaminated by an allergen such as peanut – than from airborne sources. This being said, there are also several anecdotal instances of reactions having been reported to nuts on board aeroplanes, although at the moment it is hard to say definitively what the specific trigger might have been.

For my part, I am on the side of sitting 'somewhere in between'. I find the anxiety of flying such that I feel much more comfortable picking an airline that has an active policy not to serve nuts if someone with an allergy is on-board. I'm more concerned about those little packets of nuts that everyone opens at once with a drink, than the odd person eating granola. I also take great comfort in airlines that make 'nut allergy announcements' – where the cabin crew will ask people to refrain from eating them for the duration of the flight. Even if someone in Row 27 tucking into a Snickers poses next to no risk to my child in Row 8, it feels like a signal that at least the airline is taking the issue of allergies seriously, and that is reassuring.

If I'm honest, the science may not wholly back me up on this, but it comes into the area of allergies that is all about quality of life and reduction of anxiety, and that really isn't to be sniffed at. Removing nut snacks from planes also reduces the risks of surface contamination. We've been on plenty of flights where I've found nuts and nut crumbs gathering in the creases of the seat, or whole ones rolling around the floor. They won't be removed completely because people will always snack on nuts, but any reduction feels good.

There is also a caveat in that the focus on nuts completely ignores all other allergens. Is there a danger that planes banning nuts will, as a consequence, take the focus off those with other allergies? For us, sesame or egg on a plane seat are just as much of an issue as nuts. What about those with allergies to fish, for instance; or milk?

Checklist for flying

There are a few simple steps you can take to prepare for any flight. Here goes:

Before you book

- Find out your airline's allergy policy. There is no standard 'rule', so airlines vary. The Anaphylaxis Campaign has a handy guide to various airline policies here or you should be able to find the information you need on the airline's own website.
- If relevant to you, ask whether they serve nuts on board, or will make an allergy announcement.
- Ask whether they serve any allergy-friendly food or snacks – while I would caution against eating airline food, some do serve pre-packed meals and snacks (such as British Airways' hook-up with Marks & Spencer) and there may also be fresh fruit available.
- Check whether the airline you are thinking of booking actually operates your flight – some franchise out flights to other airlines, which may not have the same allergy policies.

When you've booked

- Ask the airline to note down your child's name, booking reference and a list of their allergies. Ask for this information to be forwarded to the flight crew.
- Check whether the airline or airport require any information in advance – a doctor's letter, for instance, or proof that your medication has been prescribed.
- If you receive written assurances of any extra accommodations from the airline, print them out and take them with you when you fly.

When you arrive at the airport

- Make sure your medication and any safe snacks or food that you need are accessible in your hand luggage, along with documentation such as allergy action plans or doctor's letters.

- The 100ml liquids rule for hand luggage does not apply to medication, such as antihistamine, but you may need to show your prescription or written proof. The BSACI has a downloadable document that your doctor will need to sign. Find it at <https://www.bsaci.org/professional-resources/resources/paediatric-allergy-action-plans/>.
- The 100ml rule doesn't apply to baby milks or sterilized water (as long as you are travelling with the baby) although you will need to have any bottles available for inspection.
- Make sure you have packed enough food for snacks at the airport, if needed, as well as for the flight and taking into account any potential delays.
- On arrival, remind the airline staff at check-in about your child's allergies and check that this is noted on the system for the cabin crew.
- Ask if they will allow you to have priority early boarding so you can clean down your child's seats.

At the gate

- Get to the gate early and introduce yourself to the desk, reminding them about your child's seat number and allergies.
- Ask if they can give you priority boarding to wipe down the seat.
- Ask if they can get a message reminder to the cabin crew.

On boarding

- When you board the plane, introduce yourself and your child, and remind them of his or her allergies.
- If you have requested an in-flight announcement and no nuts to be served, remind them of this.

- If you are dealing with other allergies, quickly outline the risks – milk, cooking fish, bread with sesame and so on.
- Use wet wipes to clean down the chair, armrests, table and any other 'touch points'. An ordinary wet wipe is fine.
- Give your child's hands a quick clean once they are settled. And ... breathe.

During the flight

- Avoid using airline blankets and pillows, as they are often not washed between flights.
- Wash hands before eating.
- Don't take any unnecessary risks with foods, or try any new foods while flying.
- Make sure your medication is to hand and, if needed, use it promptly and alert the crew immediately.

According to gov.uk, when travelling with a baby you can take enough baby food, baby milk and sterilized water for the journey. There is no legal limit to how much you can take – although it's good advice to check with your airport before you travel.

You can carry breast milk in hand luggage, provided it isn't frozen. This is only permitted in the hold. Individual containers of breast milk must hold no more than 2,000ml.

Calum Smillie, now 25, was diagnosed with multiple allergies at the age of 7. He talks about his travelling experiences:

'I've travelled extensively, but I always make sure I have all my medication and it's in date. I speak to my doctor and take more EpiPens than normal. I check out where I am going beforehand and make all the necessary phone calls or send an email before leaving

home. *Some airlines are also better than others. I always travel with airlines that have a good allergy policy rather than risking it.*

I never eat any food on a plane. I bring my own and usually eat it before boarding. When I board I notify the cabin crew about my allergies and tell them what seat I'm sitting in. I always try and book a seat as close to the front of the aircraft as possible and only fly with airlines that make an announcement to the other passengers.

I used to use a cross-body bag, but now I put all my meds in a rucksack. I also favour shorts with large pockets if I'm abroad. When I travel I have bags that can keep my EpiPens at a controlled temperature and I do tend to keep everything together.

I always wear allergy wristbands when travelling and even have them printed up in the language of the country I am visiting.'

The charity MedicAlert keeps a record of your medical condition, medication, emergency contacts and any other important information. As a member, you receive one of their items of MedicAlert jewellery – a wristband, document holder or bracelet – which is embossed with your child's condition ('nut allergy', for instance) and a 24/7 helpline number that allows emergency professionals to access your most crucial information. Visit <medicalert.org.uk> for details.

There are a number of In Case of Emergency (ICE) apps also available for download to mobile phones, which work in a similar way.

19

The path to independence

Think 'teen' and a horror show of images may well flash through your mind – drunken nights, messy takeaways, kissing strangers. But all the gentle prep you've done over the years will stand your child in good stead to handle their own allergies as they hit adolescence and beyond.

That's not to say it isn't a vulnerable time. Young people aged between 16 and 24 are recognized as being at most risk of anaphylaxis. As the Anaphylaxis Campaign notes: 'This may in part be due to a decrease in parent support as they reach adulthood, more risk-taking including experimenting with new foods, travelling alone or with friends, reluctance to share information and resistance to carrying an AAI on them at all times.'

A Youth Survey carried out by the charity found 44 per cent of 15 to 25-year-olds admitted to not always carrying their AAI. But, in a systematic review by the European Academy of Allergy and Clinical Immunology (EAACI) into the challenges faced by adolescents with allergies, Vazquez-Ortiz et al[1] note: 'The period from adolescence to young adulthood offers a great opportunity, in additional to the challenges, for education, motivated by a desire for personal independence. Self-management skills learnt at this age can support the patient throughout adulthood.' They suggest that lack of knowledge is often the biggest barrier, and that 'communication [and] supportive environments' as a

---

1 'Understanding the challenges faced by adolescents and young adults with allergic conditions: A systematic review', Vazquez-Ortiz et al, *Allergy*, 2020. See: <https://pubmed.ncbi.nlm.nih.gov/32141620/>

whole were linked with better self-management. The authors added: 'Knowledge needs to be transferred to new friends and new social contexts.'

Solid peer support can indeed be hugely beneficial – having even just one competent and confident friend. A review of 'The psychosocial impact of adolescent food allergy'[2] by Cummings et al suggested: '... a good peer support network may have protective factors for adolescents with food allergy, potentially leading to fewer reactions caused by risk-taking behaviour'. And in a 2020 EAACI paper, G. Roberts et al[3] note: 'It is not that adolescents choose to engage in risks but, rather, they are willing to gamble when they lack complete knowledge. When adolescents meaningfully understand a risky situation, there are even more risk-averse than adults.'

A word of reassurance: the vast majority of parents of allergic teenagers and young adults that I have spoken to say their sons and daughters have taken their responsibilities seriously – and that, by and large, their friends have too. Equally, don't feel you need to turn a corner in a flash and suddenly let your teenager go romping over the hills of life without you. They will still need your support, and you are not doing anything wrong if they struggle from time to time. As clinical psychologist Dr Mary Halsey notes: 'Teenagers are still children and they are still going to need guidance, and still need you.'

---

2 'The psychosocial impact of food allergy and food hypersensitivity in children, adolescents and their families: a review', Cummings et al, *Allergy*, 2010. See: <https://onlinelibrary.wiley.com/doi/10.1111/j.1398-9995.2010.02342.x>

3 'EAACI Guidelines on the effective transition of adolescents and young adults with allergy and asthma', Roberts et al, *Allergy*, 2020. See: <https://onlinelibrary.wiley.com/doi/full/10.1111/all.14459>

Transition to adult allergy care

There will come a point at which your child will need to move from paediatric allergy services to adult, and it's a move that can feel very daunting – sometimes possibly more for the parent than the teenager. Your child may prefer to be seen in a more grown-up environment as they get older, and be ready for that move. Or they may equally be nervous about the prospect of handling appointments alone. The transition usually happens around the age of 16.

Some paediatric allergy clinics now provide a transition process, which begins at 13 or 14. Your child's allergy specialist may start to talk about the move, and to encourage your child to have some of their appointment time without you. They may be introduced to doctors and nurses from the adult allergy team. If this service isn't offered by your clinic, start discussing the transition with your child as they hit their teenage years, and allow them to take gradually more control over their appointments: preparing their own questions to ask in advance, having time alone with their doctor, making some of their own decisions. It will feel hard, but it's vital prep for their self-management in the future.

What's important above all, as the Children and Young People's Allergy Network Scotland (CYANS) notes, is that a young person:

- Knows their diagnosis – which foods they are allergic to, or what other allergic conditions they may have (hay fever, asthma, eczema). It may be useful to repeat allergy testing or oral food challenges at this point to confirm or rule out any uncertain diagnoses.
- Knows their prognosis – is it likely the allergy will persist? Is there any prospect for immunotherapy? Might more allergies develop?

- Knows how to keep safe – knows what to avoid, and how; can read labels; understands what constitutes safe food prep; can speak out about their allergies and understand how co-factors such as stress, alcohol, recreational drugs, lack of sleep can raise risk.
- Knows how to recognize and treat allergic reactions – knows their symptoms and when and how to use their medication, and how to show others.
- Minimizes the impact of allergy on their quality of life – can advocate for themselves, prepare and shop for their own food, manage anxiety, knows where to seek information.

They should also know how to make appointments and who to contact if symptoms change or increase. As Roberts et al note in the EAACI task force paper: 'Adolescents and young adults are more likely to follow treatment plans and attend adult service appointments when they have a good knowledge of their disease and the reasons for treatment, and good family support.'

Get support

Having a strong peer support network is key. As your child starts to go out independently, you might want to encourage them to train their friends in how to use their AAI and explain what signs and symptoms to look out for. In counteracting the fear of being 'different', it may help your child to know there are other young people going through the same journey. Some great allergy advocates include Dan Kelly, whose blog and podcast (<may-contain.com>) is all about 'breaking the stigma' of allergy and anaphylaxis. Lindiwe Lewis of <theallergytable. co.uk> is another blogger who focuses on the positive side of life with allergy.

If you can access any support groups I wholeheartedly recommend them. The Anaphylaxis Campaign sometimes runs sessions for teenagers and their parents, so do seek them out. For older teens they also have a closed – but monitored – Facebook group, specifically for 18 to 25-year-olds to chat about allergy issues. You can find it at <www.facebook.com/groups/acyoungsupportgroup/>.

Ask your allergy clinic if they run or can recommend any useful support groups. I remember vividly, when my son was first diagnosed, going to an Anaphylaxis Campaign support group where a 14-year-old boy was there with his mum, talking about how they had handled his allergies through childhood and school. He was a strapping lad, confident and comfortable, and I can't tell you the relief at seeing an actual grown boy with multiple severe allergies looking, well, alive. And happy.

That boy and his Mum were Calum and Sara Smillie. Calum, now in his twenties, who we met earlier, was seven when he was diagnosed with multiple food allergies following an anaphylactic reaction to nuts. He is now past university, with multiple trips abroad under his belt, and is well into the world of work. I asked Sara how she navigated the years from the early teens and beyond:

From what age did you start increasing Calum's independence around his allergies?

He started carrying his own medication at the age of eight. We bought him a cross-body bag that was very sporty-looking and we called it his 'nut bag'. He hung lots of badges and key chains from it and we always knew where it was.

He didn't leave the house without it. He took it to the side of the playing field when playing sport and everyone always knew to check that Calum had his 'nut bag'. I also always carried an EpiPen and his school nurse had one in her office. He didn't carry his medication at school until he was 11.

How did you handle educating friends, and parents, once Calum hit secondary school?

Whenever his friends came to our house we would practise using expired EpiPens on oranges. I remember dropping him and three friends to the cinema together for the first time. They were around 12. Before they left home, I gave them all a lesson in using the EpiPen and we explained what symptoms to look out for. They listened intently and on the way in the car I overheard them saying, 'Let's not have anything to eat so Calum stays safe.' Those boys are Calum's friends to this day.

Was Calum ever shy or anxious around his allergies?

Calum was quite a shy boy, but when he was about ten he gave a 'show and tell' talk at school to his class about his allergies, and he became a lot less anxious about telling people. I do believe that telling his classmates about his allergies when they were all in a group worked in a very positive way.

When did Calum first buy or order food for himself?

From the age of eight we encouraged him to read packaging and he ordered from restaurants with us from the age of ten. The first restaurant that he went to with his friends was Pizza Express, around the age of 14. He already knew what was safe to eat, but he also told the waiter, and in his speech to the waiter he always asked if they would inform the chef as well. We never allowed him to order a meal without saying his little speech. Every single time. He still does it. It's imperative that they never become lazy or complacent about their allergies.

How did you handle relationships and first kisses?

With Calum's allergies – and there are many – we were always quite light-hearted and, when he was younger, often said that he would have to ask a girl if she'd just had a peanut butter sandwich before he kissed her. By starting to say things like this when he was young it became something he knew about.

Similarly, how have you handled the issue of alcohol?

When he was old enough I did my research and found out which alcohol contained his allergens and printed the sheet off and we taped it inside a cupboard door.

What top tips would you give to an allergy parent facing the transition to teen years?

Make sure they know exactly what to do in every situation before they hit their teens – then it's already part of their daily life. Carrying their EpiPens, telling their friends, telling waiting staff, checking food packaging and never being afraid to say 'no' to food. One other thing we have always told Calum is that allergies are really not that bad! There are so many people out there with worse things going on and, as long as he is responsible, vigilant and careful, he can live a full, varied and fulfilling life.

And what hurdles should they look out for?

Missing out on treats is often seen as a hurdle, but make it into a positive. When Calum was younger and couldn't have some treat that everyone else was having, we gave him a pound and he saved all of his pounds up and we took him to the Chelsea FC store and he bought a Chelsea strip. This made Calum feel he wasn't missing out and, in the end, even his brother wanted a pound instead of a cake.

Calum's top tips

'Communication is the key; chat to your child about their allergies but don't make it into a big deal. Teach them how to handle situations and not to be afraid of their allergies.

My parents did the role play before every meal out. I would practise my piece and then when ordering I would say: "I am allergic to all nuts and peanuts and soya. Please can you tell the chef." They of course also chatted to the waiter but this taught me not to be afraid to speak up.

From the age of about 16, when flying my parents always made me board first and tell the crew about my allergies. They would then chat to the crew and confirm with them that they had understood all about my allergies and were going to make a PA. All of these little scenarios with my parents present gave me confidence.

Parents will always be anxious but please don't let your children hear you stressing and don't talk about your anxieties in front of them. Try to remain positive and always encourage them to try everything. I did the Duke of Edinburgh award even though I'm allergic to grass, I had to take lots of antihistamine as well as my inhaler but I managed. I played in all the football teams, I went on school trips, we just made sure that everything was well planned in advance.' – Calum Smillie, 25

It's a bumpy road

Amid all this great advice, one thing is worth keeping in mind: it won't all flow smoothly in one lovely learning curve. But don't let that get you down.

Sarah Chapman's son Will, now an adult, was diagnosed with multiple allergies at 18 months. She says: 'The preparation for adult life is not a straight line. There was a time when Will had clusters of reactions and so we stepped dramatically back as much as possible to reduce stress. During these years he also developed or redeveloped previously outgrown allergy. The hormones during teen years have impact on allergy status, so there are ups and downs. Whatever age you are at in the journey to independence, I'd say "don't panic" if you worry you've missed something, or need to catch up – think of where you are as "working towards". You'll get there.'

What if my child is shy or lacking in self-confidence?

If your child is struggling to have the confidence to speak up – for example, when eating out – Dr Mary Halsey advises trying the 'gradual exposure ladder' technique touched on in Chapter 17.

Start small, with your child observing you asking for allergy information, and talk to them about what they would ask. You might build to them next time asking for the allergy menu, and proceed up the 'rungs' after that. The older they are, the more you can encourage them to come up with the steps on the ladder themselves.

'Use as many opportunities as you can, and each time they will be gaining confidence,' adds Dr Halsey. 'Perhaps role play, and help them feel confident in the content of what they are asking and then saying it. Just get practising. If they are struggling, be low key – "oh, could you just ask for the allergy menu when the waiter comes back?" You might even ask them to pop into a café on the way to somewhere else, and say, "I'll come back later but could I just have a quick look at the allergy menu?" '

Starting these conversations early gives them plenty of time to build on their skills and confidence. Dr Halsey also suggests giving them motivation to learn: 'Tell them, we're doing this so you can go out with your friends and I don't have to come with you all the time.'

The Anaphylaxis Campaign has produced a powerful campaign film, #takethekit, to alert severely allergic young people to the importance of carrying their adrenaline auto-injector. Find it at <www.anaphylaxis.org.uk/campaigning/takethekit/>.

Romance

This is one that parents often cringe about, but if you start the conversation lightly, early on, they will know the score by the time those hormones kick in.

The problem is that allergens can remain in the saliva for anything between two and 24 hours, and even brushing teeth may not get rid of them completely. It's worth knowing that waiting several hours after eating a culprit food, and eating a non-allergenic meal or snack after that, can help to reduce the amount of allergen.

We started the chat fairly young, relating to family members – saying it's best not to kiss other people if you don't know what they have eaten. It was a handy one to raise when my son and his sister were small and biting one another became a fun game.

Sarah Chapman raised the issue of kissing with her son, Will, as part of a general discussion: 'I started with conversation about consent and added the kissing issue.' In a bid to raise awareness that casual clinches might not be a great idea – at least not without checking food status first – she says: 'I tended to talk in terms of a relationship "with someone you really like".'

Alcohol

Alcohol poses a bit of a worry on a few fronts: not only can it lower the body's threshold for severe allergic reactions (as can other factors including exercise, lack of sleep and stress), but being under the influence can blunt vigilance and lead people to take more risks.

There's also the issue of food allergens in some alcoholic drinks. Just as with food products, if any of the 14 major allergens are present they will be listed in the ingredients. The only exception is when nuts are used for distilling spirits – for example some gins use almonds as part of the process. In these cases nuts do not have to be declared on the label, because they are unlikely to trigger an allergic reaction. While risks may be small, though, it may best to play it safe. It may be a good plan to ring drinks manufacturers to check.

Common allergens in alcohol include milk in cream liqueurs, cereals containing gluten in beers and ciders, and sulphites in wine. You may also find soy sauce in Bloody Mary cocktails, aquafaba made from chickpea in vegan cocktails, and egg in drinks ranging from Gin Fizz to Advocaat. Sometimes egg, milk or fish may be used in the production of wine – but these must be declared in any vintage produced after 2012.

Another thing to think about is cross contamination at the bar – you want to be sure blenders, shakers and glassware are all thoroughly cleaned and the bartender hasn't contaminated their hands by serving nut snacks, for example. As a general rule, the simpler the better – perhaps compile a list of the brands and varieties you know are safe and stick to those (while still always reading the label).

Condoms

Oh, yay, another awkward conversation to have with your teenager. It's worth knowing that casein, a milk protein, is used in the manufacture of some condoms, with localized allergic reactions having been reported in the past. It's a good idea to contact individual condom manufacturers to check which brands may be milk-free.

Uni life

If you've done all the prep we've spoken about so far, your child's move away from home will be something they are well able to cope with.

As always, pre-planning is key. When choosing a university, have a chat with staff about any allergy procedures and policies they may have. And have a good think about what suits you when it comes to living and eating arrangements. You may opt for campus life, in self-catering or catered accommodation, or even a rented room or flat nearby.

Many students with allergies choose self-catering as it gives them more control over what they eat and when. Some universities might provide a mini fridge for personal use if you have concerns about shared kitchens, and even an extra storage cupboard for your son or daughter's room. In any event, it's important to have your own cooking equipment and utensils to keep the risks of cross contamination low. Other things you should consider include:

- Speak to the catering manager in the university canteen to find out what meals might be possible.
- Label all your food and equipment stored in shared areas.
- Tell all housemates and friends about your allergies, how to spot symptoms, what to do if you have a reaction and how to use your AAI.
- You might want to put a poster up in any shared kitchen to remind people to clean up after cooking or eating food, along with an emergency allergy action plan too.

Dan Kelly, whose blog and podcast <may-contain.com> talks about life as a young man with multiple nut allergies, went to Huddersfield University. He recalls: 'I spoke about it with Mum before I went and decided I'd go for self-catering because I could manage the food. I felt I'd be less anxious and have more control. If I did ever eat at the canteen I'd keep it really simple, like a jacket potato and tuna. I also made people aware from day one that I had a nut allergy, and that it was very serious and not just being 'fussy'. I was a bit concerned because we all know students can be messy but I made it really clear if they were going to cook with nuts then to clean up after themselves. Everyone was understanding.'

The Anaphylaxis Campaign has a helpful guide for first-time students, which you can download at <https://www.anaphylaxis.org.uk/wp-content/uploads/2019/06/Preparing-for-and-managing-your-allergies-at-university-booklet.pdf>.

Lindiwe Lewis, 29, allergy advocate and founder of The Allergy Table blog, answers some questions on growing up with allergies to nuts, sesame, legumes, kiwi, shellfish and more:

What would you advise parents to make sure their child knows before they hit the teenage years?

Boundaries – knowing it's OK to say no. My mother made me aware of all the possible situations I might get into when I became a teenager. Nothing was off-limits because she wanted me to be prepared in any situation. We discussed parties, drinking, sex, friendships, smoking, drugs ... We had an understanding that she would never judge me but she wanted me to make sure I knew how to handle anything I might come across.

You've talked about having a positive mindset to help you – what do you mean?

You can't have a positive life with a negative mind. So I catch myself when I'm talking negatively about my allergies – instead of saying, 'I don't want to go out because I can't eat, I'll get so many questions and then I'll always be "the allergy girl",' I say 'I want to see my friends and create experiences. I'll eat before going out so I save money, I won't have to worry about my allergies so I can be present with my friends and I'll have an amazing time.' That one switch can change your whole evening.

How can parents help with that?

When your child is being negative about their allergies, try saying, 'I completely understand why you feel that way, but how could we make this situation a positive one?' You might get an eye roll but if you do this all the time, it seeps in and will question their way of thinking.

Has having allergies ever stopped you from doing anything?

Not really. If I want to do something I'll do it. Only in that I won't eat at certain restaurants, or if my friends make me something I'm not sure about. There is always a way around it, you just have to ask and plan and prepare!

What do you think are the main issues to look out for as a teenager growing up with allergies?

Alcohol – not only the allergens in alcohol but the fact that it lowers inhibitions and makes everyone do things that they wouldn't do sober. Drinking from someone else's cups, eating food without checking the ingredients, kissing ... My tips: always pour your own drink (or go with the person who has offered to get you one); if you leave your cup unattended, get a new one; drink alcohol that you know is safe; and one person that goes out with you needs to know what to do in the case of a reaction – oh, and always carry your injectors (two of them)!

Did you train your friends in how to handle your allergies?

I always had someone I went out with know the signs of my reactions and how to use the EpiPen, and my only rule going out is that no one leaves without telling me.

Is it possible to travel as a young adult with allergies?

Yes! Travel, travel, travel! A lot of people travel the world for the cuisine, I get that. But you can get world food anywhere, especially in the UK. What you can't get at home is the pyramids, the Taj Mahal, the dolphins, the ruins. Don't let allergies hold you back: you can react at home, so why are you letting your allergies prevent you from seeing the wonders?

Dan Kelly, 28, was diagnosed with multiple nut allergies at the age of five. His blog and podcast may-contain.com campaigns to break the stigma around allergy.

'I started taking on responsibility when I was 14 or 15, and going out with my friends to the cinema or park. I got practice pens from the Anaphylaxis Campaign and I would practise on myself so I'd feel comfortable doing it. It helps stop you feeling anxious.

I've had such a positive experience from speaking about my allergies, nine times out of ten people are intrigued and want to know more about it. The other day I was on the Tube next to a guy I thought was eating peanuts, and I asked him if he minded not eating them because I had a severe allergy. And he was really interested – "oh, do you have an EpiPen? Can I see it?" I always say bring it up and own it!

I think that comes down to my parents: I never felt different for having my allergies, they're just part of me. The only difference is I'd bring my own packed lunch or cake. My parents didn't over-worry and it made me feel quite confident.

When it comes to alcohol, my mum was always saying, "when you get drunk don't get a takeaway at the end of the night". I could be really, really drunk but I still wouldn't risk it. I always keep food and drinks very simple – I never eat anything new if I'm out drinking. One thing that does worry me is cocktails – I went out a few weeks back and the bar didn't have ingredients, so that concerns me. I stick to what I know.

It's so important to have the allergy conversation if you feel you're getting on well with someone and it might end up in a kiss – start that dialogue before it gets to that point. You can make a bit of a joke of it. I say, "you haven't had any nuts have you?" and they say, "er, no, why?" You could talk about what your favourite foods are – "I can't eat Indian or Chinese because I've got a nut allergy". If I felt someone didn't take it seriously then, yeah, I would walk away. It's not worth it.

I've been interrailing around Europe. I made my friends aware of the importance of the EpiPen and how to use it. It's also important to make sure friends know what to do in that situation. If people start getting worked up it gets you worked up and you don't know if it's an allergic reaction or a panic attack. So I say, "stay calm, check me, see if I've got a rash and use the pen if I'm having trouble breathing". I ate a lot of McDonald's, though. There's a running joke, "Dan can go to McDonald's"; that was my comfort blanket.

To a parent, the one thing I'd say is even if you feel really anxious, try not to give off that energy. Try to make your kid feel confident and empowered. That positivity and calm helps.

You can live a very normal life with allergies, you can still go out with friends, have nights out, live abroad. It's not going to define you. But always carry your pens!'

20

Eczema and other allergic issues

Food allergies often go hand-in-hand with other atopic conditions, including hay fever, asthma and eczema.

When managing food allergies, keeping on top of these other issues is vital – for example, broken skin is more easily sensitized (see Chapter 5), or may make contact reactions more severe; uncontrolled asthma can be a factor in the severity of anaphylaxis reactions; and persistent hay fever can greatly disrupt a child's sleep and daily life.

Eczema

Eczema is a dry skin condition that causes the skin to become itchy, dry, cracked and sore. You may also hear it referred to as 'atopic dermatitis'. Sometimes this can be limited to small patches, but for others it may be more widespread. It can be incredibly itchy, which can cause a child to scratch – and, in turn, the skin can become more inflamed and sometimes even bleed.

More often than not, it develops in children before their first birthday. It tends to be a long-term condition, but it can improve or even clear completely in some children as they get older. With the appropriate treatment, it can usually be kept very well under control and may only rear its head with the occasional flare-up.

Without the proper treatment, there is a risk that the condition may worsen, and the skin may become increasingly broken, which can lead to infection.

What does it look like?

On lighter skins, eczema inflammation can appear pinkish-red and bumpy, whereas on darker skins it may present as darker brown, purplish or grey.

In infants, it may begin on the scalp and cheeks, and could be mistaken for, or associated with, cradle cap, a common condition in babies. A sign that it may be linked to food allergy is whether it is early onset, and persistent – this typically means it will arise before three to six months.

It can affect the insides of the elbows, backs of knees and face and scalp. In older babies, it may break out in chubby folds, such as the nappy area or neck. It can also present on the front of the knees, the ankles and back of elbows, as well as in the creases. There are different types of eczema, so it may look like roundish patches of inflamed skin, or fine bumps or 'dots' across the chest and tummy. The biggest clue is whether it is itchy as well as whether the skin is dry, and it can be scaly. Over time, it can become thickened or darkened ('hyperpigmented'). Scratching in response to the itch may, in fact, cause many of these skin changes.

The itch may develop over time, and babies may be seen to squirm or try to reach the offending area. If it becomes infected, it may look red and weepy or crusty, or there may be small blisters. You will need to see your GP as this may require antibiotics or, occasionally, in-hospital treatment.

How do I treat it?

The first step is to see your GP, who will be able to prescribe emollients (specially formulated moisturizers) and, where necessary to reduce inflammation, topical steroids.

Eczema can be mild, moderate or severe and some children may require more complex creams and treatments, so you may also be referred to a dermatologist specializing in skin conditions. NICE guidelines recommend referral where management has not controlled the eczema satisfactorily, or it is significantly affecting the child's sleep or behaviour.

It may take you a while to find an emollient that suits your child's skin – this is often a case of trial and error. Some may find that richer, heavier ointments work well, while others will prefer lighter creams. We tried several, with some even seemingly aggravating our son's skin, before settling on a lotion that did the trick. We also mixed it up a little – a thicker cream in the winter and a lighter one in the summer, when his skin would 'sweat' beneath anything too heavy.

Advice from the British Association for Dermatologists (BAD) is that 'the best one to use is the greasiest one you are prepared to apply'. If it proves too much by day, it may work to use a lighter version in the daytime and a greasier one at night. There is some promising new research on emollients called trilipid creams – which are similar to the skin's own natural lipid composition. Studies are ongoing.

Your child's moisturizers will be available on prescription and should be used regularly – even when their skin is 'clear', as it helps to ward off potential flare-ups. Generally speaking, you will need to reapply the creams every three or four hours where possible.

Children's allergy specialist Dr Lauri-Ann Van der Poel says: 'The cornerstone of treatment for eczema is "moisturize, moisturize, moisturize". We often find in clinic that children are just not being moisturized enough – four to six times a day, as much as you can. Not only are you keeping the skin moisturized but you are helping to maintain the skin barrier, which forms part of the body's first defence immune function. If you have eczema it is much easier for your skin to become infected or inflamed but also there is more potential for developing food allergies though skin exposure, so moisturizing is a protective measure.'

Always wash your hands before applying. Then plop large blobs of emollient on your child's skin a few centimetres apart, and smooth – rather than rub – it in, using downward strokes. If using a tub rather than a pump dispenser, use a clean spoon or spatula to avoid contamination.

You may also be prescribed a topical steroid, which is a treatment to keep swelling, redness and inflammation in check. These are creams, gels or ointments that come in varying strengths, with hydrocortisone being the mildest version. They should be used under the guidance of your doctor because the best treatment needs to be tailored in terms of the right strength and duration to deal with the eczema thoroughly.

You may have heard concerns around topical steroids 'thinning' the skin, but, as the National Eczema Society points out, topical steroids have been in use for more than 50 years and were previously used on children in much greater quantities and strengths than they are now: 'Much of the current concern about skin thinning is based on history rather than on how children are treated today.' They add: 'Parents and carers who do not use the prescribed topical steroid because of fears of skin thinning, may unwittingly be prolonging the inflammation of the skin and causing needless distress to the child. Scratching and rubbing are almost inevitable if eczema is left untreated and both can cause long-term damage to the skin.'

Official BAD guidance also notes: 'Used appropriately, topical steroids are very effective and safe to use.' Problems arise when they are used inappropriately – for too long, on the wrong part of the body, or in too potent strengths. They conclude: 'Insufficient treatment with topical steroids is generally considered by doctors to be more of a problem than overuse.'

Our dermatologist described the use of topical steroids as 'fire-fighting' – treating the first signs of a flare-up with a tiny amount, thus preventing any further outbreak. It's important to continue to apply the steroids until the active inflammation has cleared. Dr Van der Poel adds: 'One of the commonest problems is people stop too soon and they get a flare-up again quickly.' Practical advice might be to continue treatment for, or reduce it over, the same number of days after the skin has cleared as it took from starting treatment for the skin to clear. Using moisturizers frequently throughout and after helps to keep the flare-ups away for longer.

Sometimes, non-steroid anti-inflammation creams, called 'calcineurin inhibitors' are useful to control eczema when steroids are not working, or on the thinner skin of the eyelids and face.

Other treatments include 'wet wrapping' – a way of cooling the skin and providing relief. Both of these should only be used after assessment by a specialist.

What about washing?

There is a 'sweet spot' for bathing children with eczema. Too much water can be drying, but a short daily bathe using tepid or warm water and a special bath emollient – ask your doctor to prescribe one or advise you – can be very helpful and soothing.

Avoid bubble baths and regular soaps, as these will aggravate the skin. If you don't have a bath emollient, you could apply your child's medical moisturizer all over their body and let them soak and rinse off in the bath. Just beware that these creams can make them very slippery!

Pat rather than rub your child dry afterwards and reapply their usual emollient.

Beware 'natural' creams

There are many 'natural' dry skin creams on the market, but these may not be suitable for your child – and may even exacerbate their eczema. If your child has food allergies, there is also a significant risk of sensitization when using products containing common allergens, for example nut or sesame oils.

Olive oil is also not recommended as it has been found to disrupt the skin's natural barrier. Certain creams marketed as 'herbal' may even illegally contain undeclared powerful steroids. The British Association of Dermatologists says: 'It is recommended that "natural" herbal creams are not purchased as they can cause irritation and allergic reactions. Some so-called "natural" creams have been shown to contain potent steroids. Other herbal creams have been shown to contain high levels of harmful bacteria including MRSA, which may cause skin infections and septicaemia.'

What can make eczema worse?

The triggers that cause eczema to flare may be different from child to child, but generally they may include:

- extremes of heat or cold – for example, you may find that wintertime sees a flare-up, with the combination of cold outdoor temperatures and dry, centrally-heated homes and schools;
- irritants such as detergents, soaps, bubble baths and perfumed products;
- chlorine in water – after swimming, shower your child straight away and apply their usual emollients;
- scratchy fabrics like wool, or synthetics;
- food allergies;
- environmental allergens such as dust mite, pollen or animal dander;
- viral or bacterial infections.

More top tips

- Try to keep their bedroom cool.
- Stick to light cotton clothes and bedsheets where possible.
- Sleepsuits with mitts can help to stop babies scratching, and

for older children a pair of soft gloves or socks on the hands can also help at nighttime.

• Keep fingernails short.

For more information see the British Association of Dermatologists at <bad.org.uk>, the National Eczema Society at <eczema.org> and online resources at <allergyuk.org>.

Asthma

Asthma is a common lung condition, where the airways are sensitive and become inflamed and narrow when exposed to certain triggers – such as pollution, smoke, dust mites or exercise. It usually starts in childhood although can develop at any age. While it cannot be cured, it can be very well controlled with a proper management plan: the commonest reason for asthma flares is not taking the inhaler medication regularly.

What are the symptoms?

Symptoms vary between individuals and they may also come and go. The charity Asthma UK outlines some key symptoms to look out for:

• a cough that won't go away, or keeps coming back;
• a nighttime or early morning cough;
• a cough after exercise;
• a wheeze – which is a whistling or crackling sound when they breathe;
• a tight chest, which a child may describe as a 'tummy ache';
• breathlessness – look for fast breathing, or shoulders shrugging up and down.

How to get a diagnosis

Make an appointment with your GP as soon as possible – it's OK to say you need an urgent appointment because your child isn't breathing well. Before the appointment, it might be helpful to note down symptoms and when they occur, and even to video your child when they are displaying those symptoms.

For children under five, it can be difficult to confirm an asthma diagnosis; objective tests can only be carried out when they are five or older. It may be a wheeze triggered by viruses that improves as they get older. Your GP will assess your child's symptoms and prescribe treatment, such as a reliever inhaler, if required.

Asthma tests

Children with persistent asthma symptoms over the age of five will be offered one of three tests. They are:

- Peak flow – your child blows into a small plastic tube called a peak flow meter. This measures how fast they can breathe out.
- Spirometry – your child breathes into a mouthpiece for as long and fast as they can, to measure how well their lungs are working.
- Fractional Exhaled Nitric Oxide test (FeNO) – your child will breathe out a long steady breath into a FeNO machine, which measures inflammation in airways.

Asthma plan and treatment

If asthma is confirmed, you should be given an asthma care plan for your child. This will detail any preventative treatment, and how to treat an asthma attack. You can download a plan to fill out with the help of your GP from <asthma.org.uk>.

Your child will be given a reliever inhaler – which is usually blue – to treat any symptoms. This works by opening up the airways quickly and making it easier to breathe. You may be prescribed a preventer inhaler (usually brown), which reduces swelling and inflammation in the airways. You should be given a spacer: this is a large plastic tube through which your child can breathe the inhaler dose. It helps to get the medicine straight into the lungs.

It's absolutely vital to get proper advice and training from your doctor on how and when to use your child's medication. This will help to keep any potential attacks in check. If you are at all uncertain about any aspect of their asthma care plan, seek their advice.

There are other medications that your GP may also discuss with you. For lots more information head to the Asthma UK site at <asthma.org.uk>.

Hay fever

Hay fever – otherwise known as 'allergic rhinitis' – causes symptoms such as an itchy nose, watery and red eyes, a runny or blocked nose and sneezing. It is triggered by allergens from grasses, trees and plants. Rhinitis symptoms can also be caused by other environmental allergens – such as animals (horses, dogs, cats and so on), house dust mites or certain types of mould. Symptoms may be mild or be so troublesome that they can affect a child's sleep, concentration levels and general quality of life.

Sufferers can be allergic to one or more types of pollen, so their symptoms may only arise at specific times of the year. Tree pollen, such as birch, comes out in the spring, while grass pollen may be more of a problem during the summer months.

It's usually fairly easy to get a diagnosis, based on symptoms and history, so chat to your GP or allergy specialist. They may conduct skin prick tests for certain pollens, dust mites or animal allergens, or conduct a gentle examination of the inside of the nose.

Treating hay fever

If your child's hay fever is affecting their daily life, do seek help from your GP. Left untreated, rhinitis can sometimes lead to the development of asthma.

Treatments include:

- **Antihistamines** – a dose of antihistamine may relieve symptoms on 'bad days', or if exposure to the trigger occurs or can't be avoided. In some cases, they may be advised for daily use during peak pollen season. Talk to your GP.
- **Nasal sprays** – these deliver antihistamines and/or steroids directly to the nasal passages, although these don't tend to be used under the age of four. The antihistamines can help the symptoms of itching and sneezing, while the steroids can control the inflammation in the nose and relieve eye symptoms. You will need to be shown how to use these sprays, so do consult with your doctor or nurse. The spray needs to land on the inflamed area to work. It also takes time and regular use to have an effect, so don't give up!
- **Eye drops** – if eye problems are a main symptom, regular use of prescription eye drops can help to block the release of histamine. Don't use eye drops on children without first discussing with your GP. There are newer drops – for example, Opatanol – that sting less and are more effective than older sodium cromoglicate drops, but these are only available on prescription.

Immunotherapy

Many allergy clinics provide immunotherapy treatments for children who have severe and debilitating rhinitis symptoms. This is a treatment to 'desensitize' the body so that it no longer reacts to the culprit allergen.

There are two types – subcutaneous immunotherapy (an injection) and sublingual immunotherapy (a daily tablet or spray given under the tongue). Subcutaneous immunotherapy takes place over a period of three to five years and needs to be given in a controlled medical environment. Sublingual immunotherapy, after the first dose, can continue to be given in the home. Both have proven to be very effective and to give long-lasting benefit.

Top tips

It may help to avoid exposure to your child's trigger where possible. Strategies might include:

- Stay indoors until after midday, when pollen tends to have settled.
- Avoid windy days or thunderstorms.
- Wear sunglasses to protect the eyes.
- Shower when home to wash off the pollen – or at least wash your child's face and hair if they have been playing outside.
- Stay inside when grass is being mown.
- Keep windows at home and in the car closed during peak pollen season, and particularly in the morning and early evening when pollens are released.
- If possible, consider changing your child's bedroom if the culprit plants or trees are outside their window.
- Avoid drying clothes outside when the pollen count is high.
- Use cold compresses to soothe irritated eyes (a cotton pad soaked in cool water is fine).

Keep an eye on the pollen count via <pollenuk.co.uk>, which also has a handy calendar for when different pollens are at their highest in the various regions of the UK.

The main pollen season – mainly birch and oak – runs from late March to early June, while the main grass pollen season runs from late April to July.

Animals, house dust mites and more

There are various environmental allergens alongside pollens that can trigger allergic symptoms, such as rhinitis, asthma and eczema. Among the most common are animals – typically cats, dogs or horses, although any animals (even reptiles) can cause symptoms. The allergens are found not in the animal's fur, as often thought, but in their saliva and the skin cells they shed, called dander.

There is no such thing as an 'allergen free' or 'hypoallergenic' cat or dog, although some breeds shed less dander and so are less likely to trigger a reaction. If animals shed a lot of fur or hair, that hair will have saliva or dander attached, posing an increased risk. If exposure to a pet is unavoidable, try to keep pets outside or at least out of the bedroom, do not allow them to sit on beds, cushions or sofas, wash pet bedding regularly on a hot wash, and remember to wash hands after touching or being licked by a pet. It may also be helpful to 'pre-treat' with antihistamine, preferably a long-acting, non-drowsy one such as cetirizine.

If you are considering buying a pet, it may be possible for your allergy clinic to test your child for common allergens – such as dogs, cats, horses, hamsters and guinea pigs. It is worth bearing in mind that cat dander is much finer and so a greater risk, especially to children with asthma. It also lingers: studies have shown how cat allergen can persist for up to 30 weeks in a home, even after the cat has been removed.

It might also be a sensible idea to pay regular visits to a friend or family member with a cat or dog, if you are considering welcoming one into the family. One visit is not enough to judge whether your child is allergic, as it takes time to develop an allergy. It is impossible to predict with certainty if your child will be allergic to a pet, so you should bear in mind that having to rehome a new dog or cat may unfortunately be necessary, if your child's symptoms are more than mild.

House dust mites are a very common trigger, which are notoriously difficult to tackle. These are microscopic creatures that live in the dust in our homes – their droppings are inhaled and cause allergic symptoms. Helpful tips include using allergy-proof covers on beds and washing all bedding not covered in allergen-proof covers once a week, at no less than 60 degrees.

Avoid the bottom bunk, where allergen can fall on your child. If possible, go for non-carpeted rooms, which harbour fewer dust mites. Vacuum regularly with a HEPA filter, damp wipe surfaces regularly, and wash soft toys frequently at 60 degrees – or place them in a plastic bag in the freezer for at least 12 hours, then wash on their usual gentle setting. Try to increase ventilation through windows, extractor fans and trickle vents.

Moulds also produce spores that are airborne, and can be found both indoors and outdoors, where they thrive in damp, warm conditions. Ventilation is key to controlling mould in the home.

For more information on how to manage environmental allergies, see <allergyuk.org>.

21

Where else might I find allergens?

Food and drink aside, there are other places that allergens can hide, so the cardinal rule for everything – from toiletries to medicines – is Always Read the Label.

Here's a quick guide to help you.

Toiletries and cosmetics

If you think handling food labelling is tricky, wait until you enter the mind-boggling world of cosmetic and skincare labelling.

By law, all cosmetics and toiletries (including things like toothpaste, deodorant, suncreams, moisturizers and perfumes) must list all ingredients. This used to come under the EU Cosmetics Regulation but has now been transferred into UK law. Where packaging is very small, this information has to appear on an enclosed or attached leaflet, label or tag. Some manufacturers use 'peel up' labels to reveal the full ingredients list. But they are not required to emphasize any of the '14 allergens' in food labelling law – or to list them in the same way. Instead, they have to use the so-called International Nomenclature of Cosmetic Ingredients (INCI). These apply to almost all countries in the world, with few exceptions.

For those with food allergies, it's a good idea to know the Latin as well as the English words for your allergen and its derivatives.

Health writer and co-founder of the Free From Skincare Awards, Alex Gazzola, has a few top tips and things to remember:

'Learn the Latin for your allergens, and always read the ingredients.

Generally speaking, the greater allergy risk is for "leave on" products (moisturizing creams and lotions) or things you immerse yourself in, like bath bombs, as well as eye creams and lip balms, rather than "rinse off" products (shower gel, soap).

Be cautious when using new products, as reactions may occur to non-food ingredients such as preservatives or fragrances.

Ask for recommendations from fellow allergy parents, and check brand websites. Many have allergy advice guidance sections or ingredients you can scan through.'

It's highly unlikely that 'traces' or cross contamination would be a problem with cosmetics in the same way that they are with foods, and certainly if you are dealing with a well-known, major name. Smaller, homemade brands may require greater scrutiny, so you may want to ring them to check whether there is any risk of contamination with your allergen.

Even where nut oils are used, often in cosmetics these would be so highly refined as not to pose a risk of allergic reaction – but it's best to err on the side of caution. It might be sensible to 'patch test' anything new by dabbing a little on the inside of the elbow and leaving for 24 hours. Only introduce one new product at a time.

Don't forget to watch out for things like lipsticks and cosmetics used by romantic partners, too.

Here's a handy list of some common food allergens in Latin:

Almond: *Prunus dulcis, Prunus amygdalus dulcis, Prunus amara*
Banana: *Musa sapientum, Musa paradisiacal, Musa acuminate, Musa balbisiana, Musa basjoo, Musa nana*
Brazil: *Bertholletia excelsa*
Cashew: *Anacardium occidentale*
Celery: *Apium graveolens*
Chickpea: *Cicer arietinum*
Coconut: *Cocus nucifera*

Egg: *Ovum*

Fish liver oil: *Piscum iecur*

Hazelnut: *Corylus rostrata, Corylus americana, Corylus avellana*

Kiwi: *Actinidia chinensis, Actinidia deliciosa*

Lupin: *Lupinus albus, Lupinus luteus, Lupinus texensis, Lupinus subcarnosus*

Macadamia: *Macadamia ternifolia, Macadamia integrifolia*

Milk: *Lac*

Mustard: *Brassica alba, Brassica nigra, Brassica juncea*

Oat: *Avena sativa, Avena strigosa*

Peanut: *Arachis hypogaea*

Pistachio: *Pistacia vera, Pistacia manshurica*

Rice: *Oryza sativa*

Rye: *Secale cereale*

Sesame: *Sesamum indicum*

Soya: *Glycine soja, Glycine max*

Walnut: *Juglans regia, Juglans nigra*

Wheat: *Triticum vulgare, Triticum aestivum*

Whey Protein: *Lactis proteinum*

Face paints

For kids with allergies, it's not only food-related ingredients that may cause problems, but harsh products that inflame more sensitive skin. One popular British brand that is often recommended is Snazaroo – they don't use egg, dairy or nuts, although they do use soya derivative. The American brand Kiss Freely is free from nuts, eggs, dairy, soy, wheat, sesame, shea butter, peas and more.

Medicines

Another 'always read the label' one – not only on the outer packaging, but also on the patient information leaflet inside the box. If you have been prescribed any medicine, check with the doctor, and again with the pharmacist, that it doesn't contain your allergen.

You can also check the list of ingredients for any drug that is licensed for use in the UK by visiting <medicines.org.uk> and using the 'search' bar.

Look out for allergens in unexpected places – peanut oil in vitamins, ear drops and nappy rash creams, or sesame oil in hay fever sprays. Don't assume, just check.

Unexpected allergens

Sometimes an allergen can pop up where you least expect it, so vigilance is your watchword – within reason.

As well as cosmetics, medicines and pet food, you might find nut oils in toilet paper and fabric softeners, milk or wheat in innovative compostable packaging, or even milk – yes, milk – in clothes. The high street retailer Uniqlo has a HeatTech range that contains milk protein in the fabric. Realistically, many of these products would pose minimal risk, if any, but as there is currently little research into the allergenic properties of these products, you are probably best erring on the side of caution.

There is also some scrutiny currently around novel food products – for example, there are some products catering for the plant-based market that used lab-generated proteins. One brand of ice cream – 'Perfect Day' – is made from precision fermented whey and casein. These have never been near a cow, but they are identical to those produced by the animal, so will cause identical reactions and should be avoided by anyone with a milk allergy.

22

Immunotherapy and hopes for the future

Of course, what we all want is a cure – a magic pill that will send food allergies into retreat and allow our kids to eat and live freely again. The bad news? We're not there. The good news? There are tentative steps in the right direction.

You will no doubt have read and heard about the various immunotherapy trials ongoing in the UK and internationally. Every so often a newspaper headline proclaims a 'potential cure' for food allergies, which brings fresh hope. But are these treatments available to all? Do they work? Are they suitable for my child? Here's the lowdown on what's available, and what is – and isn't – possible.

What is immunotherapy?

Immunotherapy, previously known as 'desensitization', is a medical treatment for allergies. As the Anaphylaxis Campaign puts it: 'The idea is that the patient's immune system can be "trained" to tolerate the allergen and therefore not cause allergic symptoms.'

While various immunotherapy treatments for food allergies have had success, it is not yet known whether that tolerance persists for years to come. This is because it has only really been investigated as an option over the past five to ten years, and studies have had mixed results. Consequently it cannot be seen as a 'cure', although it may increase tolerance to protect the patient from the risks of accidental ingestion.

Paediatric allergy specialist Dr Mich Lajeunesse is steering group chair of the BSACI's BRIT registry of immunotherapy treatments in the UK. He explains the difference between a 'cure' and what immunotherapy can currently achieve: 'It's important to manage expectations. A cure is taking you to a situation where you don't have a peanut allergy – you can eat a Snickers bar today and then nothing for the next 14 months, and then a peanut butter sandwich the next time and you have no problems at all. That's what a proper cure would look like. In practice, what most people are thinking is that, when you have been desensitized [through immunotherapy] you will need to be eating some form of pharmaceutical nut product or real world food in a small amount, say, every day. For example, two M&Ms instead of a tablet and you take that regularly. What "regularly" looks like we don't know at the moment.'

When successful, immunotherapy raises your threshold of tolerance, and any symptoms you may have would be milder and less likely to be a systemic allergic reaction (anaphylaxis).

Dr Lajeunesse explains: 'You would have to go out of your way to have a reaction. I think it's a game changer for many families, especially if you have only peanut allergy.' It is not yet available as a treatment on the NHS, although there is research ongoing, and there are often calls for new participants.

While there are significant hurdles to breach, not least gaining funding, and NICE approval, there are hopes that immunotherapy treatments may begin to be rolled out within the next two or three years. Dr Lajeunesse adds: 'I think we will see food allergy treatment being transformed by immuno-therapy over the next ten years. It's really going to take off.'

There are three main methods of immunotherapy:

1. Oral immunotherapy (OIT)

In oral immunotherapy, small but increasing doses of food are swallowed over a period of months, until the body is 'trained' not to react. There are ongoing studies investigating OIT's efficacy both in the UK and internationally.

It is important to note that up to 20 per cent of patients do not tolerate the treatment, and it can be gruelling: there are the logistics of frequent hospital appointments, the need to miss chunks of school and work as a consequence, and the fact that many can experience allergic reactions as they progress along the immunotherapy route. Some may experience anaphylaxis.

Studies also suggest that the effects to date have not been long-lasting: if the therapy is stopped, the allergy returns. And even when a child has been desensitized, they may still experience low grade symptoms to the 'maintenance dose'.

The UK studies involving children include:

BOPI

The Boiled Oral Peanut Immunotherapy (BOPI) research programme, at Imperial College London, uses boiled rather than roasted peanut – which researchers propose is better tolerated. Results in 2019 showed 'sustained unresponsiveness' to peanut following one year of treatment, but a further clinical trial continues.

Aimmune Therapeutics

The US-based international biopharmaceutical company Aimmune is sponsoring a number of studies in peanut immuno-therapy across the UK, using peanut protein capsules or sachets under the brand name PALFORZIA.

Two Phase III clinical trials – PALISADE and ARTEMIS – recruited more than 600 children aged four to 17 across 60 international sites, including the Evelina London, Southampton Hospital and King's College London. More than half of partic-ipants were able to tolerate the equivalent of seven to eight peanuts after nine months of treatment. An international trial is ongoing into children aged one to three.

Aimmune have submitted applications for marketing approval of their peanut-based product to US and European Medicines regulators and are currently considering extending their studies to egg allergy. While it is likely to become available in the near future, it will begin as a private treatment until – if and when – it gains NHS approval and funding.

Further information is at <aimmune.com>.

Camallergy

This is a spin-off company founded by researchers at Cambridge University Hospital's NHS Foundation Trust, which is planning to launch a peanut-based oral immunotherapy treatment – so-called 'pull-apart' peanut protein capsules.

In 2014, the team revealed results of their trials involving children with peanut allergy aged 7–16. The majority of participants were able to tolerate peanuts after the immunotherapy treatment, with further increasing levels of tolerance over time. Camallergy is now preparing for Phase III studies to confirm the results in children and possibly adults. See <camallergy.com> for details.

A private service for patients is up and running at Cambridge Peanut Allergy Clinic, based at Addenbrooke's Hospital. This is a two year programme and bears a considerable cost – upwards of £15,000. Further information is available at <cuh.nhs.uk/our-services/peanut-allergy/>.

2. Epicutaneous immunotherapy (EPIT)

The food allergen is applied to the skin via a patch or plaster. This treatment is being developed by global pharmaceutical company DBV Technologies. Their product, Viaskin, is an electrostatic patch that activates the immune system through intact skin.

The intention is that it will be self-administered, non-invasive and easy to use. Studies are ongoing to assess Viaskin for milk, egg and peanut allergy. The company says: 'Viaskin safely provides allergenic information to the immune system without entering the bloodstream. Once applied to skin, Viaskin creates a condensation chamber that hydrates the skin and solubilises the allergen, allowing it to penetrate the epidermis.'

A study assessing EPIT in peanut-allergic children is taking place in the UK. More information is at <dbv-technologies.com>.

3. Sublingual immunotherapy (SLIT)

This is similar to oral immunotherapy, except the treatment (containing the food allergen) is held under the tongue rather than swallowed.

A number of studies have been published investigating SLIT for food allergy, including to milk and peanut. While SLIT appears to be much safer than oral immunotherapy, it is also less effective, although a recent study found some benefit after three years of treatment (Kim et al, 2019).

Researchers at Imperial College London are currently investigating whether using SLIT as a pre-treatment before OIT can improve the safety of conventional immunotherapy in cow's milk allergy. The study, known as SOCMA, began in July 2018.

Other treatments

Many groups are investigating ways to improve outcomes in oral immunotherapy, predominantly for peanut allergy.

Researchers in Melbourne are looking at whether combining peanut OIT with probiotics improves treatment results, while a study led out of Sydney is assessing whether a dietary fibre supplement can have a similar effect.

A group in Boston commenced a study in June 2019 to look at whether a medicine called VE416 (which contains inactive bacteria) in combination with vancomycin (an antibiotic) can improve outcomes in oral immunotherapy for peanut. And there are various trials looking into whether biologic drugs may improve immunotherapy outcomes – including omalizumab (known under the brand name Xolair) and dupilumab (known as Dupixent).[1]

The peanut vaccine

This one has grabbed a few headlines – the prospect of a vaccine to treat those with peanut allergy. Phase I human clinical trials by UK biotech firm Allergy Therapeutics are poised to begin, following promising results from tests using mice.

The vaccine aims to work by hiding the peanut allergen in a harmless synthesized virus derived from cucumber (yes, really). The peanut protein is bound to that virus so the immune system doesn't 'see' it and trigger an allergic reaction.

Instead, it elicits a different response that generates memory cells to identify the peanut protein without the immune response. The hope is that the next time the body is exposed to the peanut it identifies it, and realizes it is not dangerous.

For information on all ongoing clinical trials see <clinicaltrials.gov>. *You may also wish to join the Anaphylaxis Campaign, which advertises many new and recruiting clinical trials and studies to its members.*

Testing

As touched on in earlier chapters, testing for food allergy remains in many ways fairly rudimentary. By this I mean that no test is categorical proof positive or otherwise, requiring a doctor

1 'Long-term sublingual immunotherapy for peanut allergy in children: clinical and immunologic evidence of desensitisation', Kim et al, *Journal of Allergy & Clinical Immunology*, 2019. See: <https://www.jacionline.org/article/S0091-6749(19)31020-6/fulltext>

to interpret those results alongside the patient's full history. In some cases a food challenge is also necessary, to confirm or rule out allergy. Neither can a test diagnose how mild or severe any future reactions might be.

But there is research ongoing into new and more sophisticated testing techniques. Among these are the Basophil Activation Test (BAT). A sample of the patient's blood is mixed with the suspected allergen, then basophils – a type of white blood cell – are analysed for the presence of a molecule known as CD63, indicating allergy. Results are available within three hours.

A recent study[2] of 92 children at Guy's and St Thomas' Hospital, London, found BAT to be highly accurate at diagnosing allergies to nuts and seeds between 96–100 per cent of the time. Professor Graham Roberts, a consultant in paediatric allergy at University Hospital Southampton, has said: 'This is exciting as a lot of the time skin prick testing and IgE tests are inconclusive.' However, because it requires blood to be taken and the tests to be run within a few hours, hospitals will need the right equipment and resources to manage this. It may also not work in all patients. Studies continue.

Other potential breakthroughs include mast cell activation testing (MAT), which uses mast cells cultured in a lab, to which the patient's blood plasma is added. This could end up being easier to use than BAT.

Meanwhile, component testing is available in some allergy clinics for a number of allergens, including peanut and hazelnut. This isolates the different proteins in an allergen. Depending on which ones the patient is sensitive to, this can better predict the likelihood of allergy as opposed to a cross-reactive reaction related to pollen. It can provide clearer information if conventional tests or a patient history are uncertain. Paediatric allergy

2 'Basophil Activation Test Reduces Oral Food Challenges to Nuts and Sesame', Santos et al, *Journal of Allergy & Clinical Immunology*, 2020. See: <https://www.sciencedirect.com/science/article/pii/S2213219820314033>

specialist Dr Mich Lajeunesse says: 'Component testing is very useful for older kids and adults when they have hay fever, because the pollen allergy can interfere with peanut allergy testing, so you get false positives. Are you allergic to the pollen protein or the seed protein? There are more component tests for different allergens coming on-stream all the time.'

The last word

It's hard to keep a sunny outlook when you're battling food allergies day-to-day. But there are positives that come from diagnosis, and the rare wisdom being an allergy parent confers. Here are some fellow allergy parents' thoughts on the plus points, to bring some cheer:

'We eat healthier just because so much is cooked from scratch, and so few fast food options are available to us.'

'Allergies mean we know exactly what goes into everything we eat.'

'It's taught us empathy – the ability to understand that everyone is dealing with something.'

'It can instil a real determination not to follow the crowd. Your life depends on your ability to advocate for yourself, to speak up and state what is and isn't safe.'

'My kids learnt to cook and adapt recipes, which is such an important life skill.'

'There's no way on earth I would have made bagels from scratch if it wasn't for allergies – and they're good!'

'An unexpected positive is my kids tell me they feel "special" – it gives them an interesting/different identity.'

'I think I'm more laid back about other risks – don't worry about climbing up that massive tree, just don't eat that sandwich.'

'Delayed gratification is a thing, for sure! My child knows sometimes he just can't have that treat, and so he might have to wait to have something else instead.'

'Amazing knowledge of food and nutrition, miles ahead of peers in school.'

'We are more mindful about food and meals. And we don't take anything for granted.'

'I think my child growing up with allergies has been a factor in her developing a can-do attitude to life.'

'It gives you a fuller appreciation of the simple things – when a meal is safe, when family can eat together, finding a safe ice cream on the beach, or that one person that goes the extra mile.'

Resources

Charities and allergy organizations

Allergy UK
01322 619898
allergyuk.org

Anaphylaxis Campaign
01252 542029
anaphylaxis.org.uk

Asthma UK
0300 222 5800
asthma.org.uk

British Society of Allergy & Clinical Immunology (BSACI)
bsaci.org

Children and Young People's Allergy Network Scotland (CYANS)
cyans.scot.nhs.uk

Natasha Allergy Research Foundation
narf.org.uk

Eczema

British Association of Dermatologists (BAD)
bad.org.uk

National Eczema Association
nationaleczema.org

Dietitians

British Dietetic Association
bda.uk.com

Training and education

Allergy Academy
allergyacademy.org
The King's College London-founded 'academy' offers courses, resources and training to healthcare professionals and parents.

Allergy Action
allergyaction.org
Head here for allergy research, training, news and information from Dr Hazel Gowland, who has had a lifelong nut allergy and is a leading expert patient and consumer advocate.

Allergy Adventures
allergyadventures.com
This little website is packed with fantastic kids' activities, school information packs and more.

AllergyWise
Allergywise.org.uk
Free and paid courses for carers, schools and healthcare professionals from the Anaphylaxis Campaign.

EpiPen
epipen.co.uk

Jext
jext.co.uk

Allergy accessories

Allergy Buddies
allergybuddies.com

Allergy Lifestyle
allergylifestyle.com

Foodie blogs

Allergy Mums
allergymums.co.uk

Glutarama
glutarama.com

Lucy's Friendly Foods
lucysfriendlyfoods.com

My Allergy Boy
myallergyboy.com

The Intolerant Gourmand
intolerantgourmand.com

The Free From Fairy
freefromfairy.com

Guidance and legislation

Food Standards Agency
food.gov.uk

NICE
nice.org.uk

Other handy websites

Allergy Insight
allergy-insight.com
A hugely knowledgeable and detailed blog on food allergy, intolerance, coeliac disease and beyond from expert health writer Alex Gazzola.

Allergic Living
allergicliving.com
The one and only comprehensive online magazine devoted to allergy. This is a Canadian site but its information and resources are relevant to all.

Kyle Dine Music
kyledine.com
Kyle is a hugely popular American food allergy educator – using puppetry, songs and more to raise awareness and confidence among kids.

The Allergy Collective
allergycollective.co.uk
A parent-run platform offering 'support and solidarity'.

The Allergy Team
theallergyteam.com
A digital platform offering webinars, meet-ups, expert Q&As and more.

North American websites

American Academy of Allergy, Asthma & Immunology
aaaai.org

American College of Allergy, Asthma & Immunology
acaai.org

Food Allergy Research and Education (FARE)
foodallergy.org

Kids with Food Allergies
kidswithfoodallergies.org

Asthma Allergies Children
asthmaallergieschildren.com

References

1 British Society for Allergy & Clinical Immunology. See: <https://www.bsaci.org/patients/ frequently-asked-questions/>

2 'Sense About Science: Making Sense of Allergies'. See: <https://archive.senseaboutscience.org/data/files/ resources/189/Making-Sense-of-Allergies.pdf>

3 'The prevalence of and risk factors for atopy in early childhood: a whole population birth cohort study', Tariq et al, *The Journal of Allergy & Clinical Immunology*, 1998. See: <https://www.jacionline.org/article/ S0091-6749(19)31020-6/fulltext>

4 'Defining challenge-proven coexistent nut and sesame seed allergy: a prospective multicentre European study', Brough et al, *The Journal of Allergy & Clinical Immunology*, 2020. See: <https://www.jacionline.org/article/%20 S0091-6749(19)31409-5/fulltext>

5 'Emergency treatment of anaphylactic reactions: Guidelines for healthcare providers', Resuscitation Council UK. See: <https://www.resus.org.uk/ library/additional-guidance/guidance-anaphylaxis/ emergency-treatment>

6 'Food anaphylaxis in the United Kingdom: analysis of national data, 1998-2018', Baseggio Conrado et al, *the BMJ*, 2021. See: <https://www.bmj.com/content/372/bmj.n733>

7 'Incidence of fatal food anaphylaxis in people with food allergy: a systematic review and meta-analysis', Umasunthar et al, *Clinical & Experimental Allergy*, 2013. See: <https://onlinelibrary.wiley.com/doi/epdf/10.1111/ cea.12211>

8 'Peanuts in the air – clinical and experimental studies', Bjorkman et al, *Clinical & Experimental Allergy*, 2021. See: <https://onlinelibrary.wiley.com/doi/10.1111/cea.13848>

9 'Fatal anaphylaxis due to transcutaneous allergen exposure: An exceptional case', Foong et al, *The Journal of Allergy & Clinical Immunology*, 2020. See: <https://www.sciencedirect.com/science/article/abs/pii/S2213219819308499?via%3Dihub>

10 'Myths, facts and controversies in the diagnosis and management of anaphylaxis', Anagnostou et al, *Archives of Diseases in Childhood*, 2019. See: <https://adc.bmj.com/content/104/1/83>

11 'The Emperor Has No Symptoms: The Risks of a Blanket Approach to Using Epinephrine Autoinjectors for All Allergic Reactions', Turner et al, *The Journal of Allergy & Clinical Immunology In Practice*, 2016. See: <https://pubmed.ncbi.nlm.nih.gov/27283056/>

12 'Using NHS Data to monitor trends in the occurrence of severe, food induced allergic reactions', Imperial College London. See: < https://www.food.gov.uk/research/food-allergy-and-intolerance-research/using-nhs-data-to-monitor-trends-in-the-occurrence-of-severe-food-induced-allergic-reactions>

13 'Auvi-Q Versus EpiPen: Preferences of Adults, Caregivers, and Children', Camargo et al, *The Journal of Allergy & Clinical Immunology In Practice*, 2013. See: <https://www.jaci-inpractice.org/article/S2213-2198(13)00125-6/fulltext

14 'Allergy: The Unmet Need – A blueprint for better patient care', Corrigan et al, *Royal College of Physicians*, 2003. See: <https://www.bsaci.org/wp-content/uploads/2020/02/allergy_the_unmet_need.pdf>

15 'A food allergy epidemic... or just another case of overdiagnosis?', R. Boyle & P. Turner, *The BMJ*, 2021. See: <https://blogs.bmj.com/bmj/2021/02/17/a-food-allergy-epidemic-or-just-another-case-of-overdiagnosis/>

16 'Prevalence and cumulative incidence of food hypersensitivity in the first 3 years of life', Venter et

al, *Allergy*, 2008. See: <https://pubmed.ncbi.nlm.nih.gov/18053008/>

17 'Food allergy in under 19s: assessment and diagnosis', NICE. See: <https://www.nice.org.uk/guidance/cg116/ifp/chapter/Person-centred-care>

18 'Specificity of allergen skin testing in predicting positive open food challenges to milk, egg and peanut in children', Sporik et al, *Clinical & Experimental Allergy*, 2000. See: <https://pubmed.ncbi.nlm.nih.gov/11069561/>

19 'Sense About Science: Making Sense of Allergies', 2015. See: <https://www.immunology.org/sites/default/files/making-sense-of-allergies.pdf>

20 'Parental anxiety before and after food challenges in children with suspected peanut and hazelnut allergy', Zijlstra et al, *Paediatric Allergy & Immunology*, 2010. See: <https://onlinelibrary.wiley.com/doi/abs/10.1111/j.1399-3038.2009.00929.x>

21 'Anxiety and stress in mothers of food allergic children', Lau et al, *Paediatric Allergy & Immunology*, 2014. See: <https://pubmed.ncbi.nlm.nih.gov/24750570/>

22 'Quality of life in the setting of anaphylaxis and food allergy', L. Lange, *Allergo Journal International*, 2014. See: < https://www.ncbi.nlm.nih.gov/pmc/articles/PMC4479473/>

23 'Prospects for Prevention of Food Allergy', Allen et al, *The Journal of Allergy & Clinical Immunology*, 2016. See: <https://pubmed.ncbi.nlm.nih.gov/26755097/>

24 'Mechanisms of food allergy', Sampson et al, *The Journal of Allergy & Clinical Immunology*, 2018. See: <https://www.jacionline.org/article/S0091-6749(17)31809-2/pdf>

25 'Prospects for Prevention of Food Allergy', Allen et al, *The Journal of Allergy & Clinical Immunology*, 2016. See: <https://pubmed.ncbi.nlm.nih.gov/26755097/>

26 'Epidemiologic risks for food allergy', G. Lack, *The Journal of Allergy & Clinical Immunology*, 2008. See:

<https://www.thelancet.com/journals/lancet/article/ PIIS0140-6736(19)32984-8/fulltext>

27 'Daily emollient during infancy for prevention of eczema: the BEEP randomised controlled trial', Chalmers et al, *The Lancet*, 2020. See: < https://www.thelancet. com/journals/lancet/article/PIIS0140-6736(19)32984-8/ fulltext>

28 'Early consumption of peanuts in infancy is associated with a low prevalence of peanut allergy', Du Toit et al, *The Journal of Allergy & Clinical Immunology*, 2008. See: <https:// pubmed.ncbi.nlm.nih.gov/19000582/>

29 'Learning Early About Peanut Allergy', Lack et al, Immune Tolerance Network. See: <http://www.leapstudy.co.uk>

30 'Effect of Avoidance on Peanut Allergy after Early Peanut Consumption', Du Toit et al, *The New England Journal of Medicine*, 2016. See: <https://www.nejm.org/doi/ full/10.1056/NEJMoa1514209>

31 'Enquiring About Tolerance (EAT) study: Feasibility of an early allergenic food introduction regimen, Perkin et al, *The Journal of Allergy & Clinical Immunology*, 2016. See: <https://www.ncbi.nlm.nih.gov/pmc/articles/ PMC4852987/>

32 'Hay fever, hygiene, and household size', D. P. Strachan, *The BMJ*, 1989. See: <https://www.ncbi.nlm.nih.gov/pmc/ articles/PMC1838109/>

33 'Pacifier cleaning practices and risk of allergy development', Hesselmar et al, *Paediatrics*, 2013. See <https://pubmed.ncbi.nlm.nih.gov/23650304/>

34 'Dog ownership at three months of age is associated with protection against food allergy', Marrs et al, *European Journal of Allergy & Clinical Immunology*, 2019. See: <https://onlinelibrary.wiley.com/doi/abs/10.1111/ all.13868>

35 'Rural and urban food allergy prevalence from the South African Food Allergy study', Botha et al, *The Journal of*

Allergy & Clinical Immunology, 2019. See: <https://www.jacionline.org/article/S0091-6749(18)31130-8/fulltext>

36 'Allergy: Policy Briefing', *British Society for Immunology*, 2017. See: <https://www.immunology.org/sites/default/files/Allergy%20briefing.pdf>

37 'Mothers who swim during pregnancy increase their child's risk of eczema and asthma, scientists warn', *Daily Mail*, 2013. See: <https://www.dailymail.co.uk/news/article-2408374/Mothers-swim-pregnancy-increase-childs-risk-eczema-asthma-scientists-warn.html>

38 'Stunted microbiota and opportunistic pathogen colonisation in caesarean-section birth', Shao et al, *Nature*, 2019. See: <https://www.nature.com/articles/s41586-019-1560-1>

39 'The hapten-atopy hypothesis III: the potential role of airborne chemicals', McFadden et al, *British Journal of Dermatology*, 2013. See: <https://onlinelibrary.wiley.com/doi/abs/10.1111/bjd.12602>

40 'Expectant mothers who swim 'may give baby asthma', *The Telegraph*, 2013. See: <https://www.telegraph.co.uk/news/health/news/10278263/Expectant-mothers-who-swim-may-give-baby-asthma.html>

41 'Grandmothers' Smoking Linked To Grandchildren's Asthma Decades Later', *Science Daily*, 2005. See: <https://www.sciencedaily.com/releases/2005/05/050505224059.htm>

42 'Food Allergy Sensitization and Presentation in Siblings of Food Allergic Children', Gupta et al, *The Journal of Allergy & Clinical Immunology*, 2016. See: <https://www.ncbi.nlm.nih.gov/pmc/articles/PMC5010481/>

43 'Food Allergy Sensitization and Presentation in Siblings of Food Allergic Children', Gupta et al, *The Journal of Allergy & Clinical Immunology*, 2016. See: <https://www.ncbi.nlm.nih.gov/pmc/articles/PMC5010481/>

44   <https://www.bsaci.org/wp-content/uploads/2020/02/
     pdf_Infant-feeding-and-allergy-prevention-PARENTS-
     FINAL-booklet.pdf>
45   'The Maternal Diet Index in Pregnancy is associated with
     offspring allergic diseases', Venter et al, *Allergy*, 2021. See:
     <https://pubmed.ncbi.nlm.nih.gov/34018205/>
46   Assessment of Evidence About Common Infant
     Symptoms and Cow's Milk Allergy', Munblit et al, *JAMA
     Paediatrics*, 2020. See: https://jamanetwork.com/journals/
     jamapediatrics/article-abstract/276408147>
47   'Food Allergy: past, present and future', H. Sampson,
     Allergology International, 2016. See: <https://www.
     sciencedirect.com/science/article/pii/S1323893016301137>
48   <https://www.newstatesman.com/ideas/2013/08/
     was-downfall-richard-iii-caused-strawberry>
49   'Sense About Science: Making Sense of Allergies',
     2015. See: <https://senseaboutscience.org/wp-content/
     uploads/2016/09/Making-Sense-of-Allergies-1.pdf>
50   <https://www.vaccinestoday.eu/faq/
     do-immunisations-cause-allergies/>
51   'Safety of live attenuated influenza vaccine in young
     people with egg allergy', Turner et al, *The BMJ*, 2015. See:
     <https://www.bmj.com/content/351/bmj.h6291>
52   <https://www.gov.uk/government/collections/
     immunisation-against-infectious-disease-the-green-
     book#the-green-book>
53   <https://www.theguardian.com/society/2019/jun/08/
     junk-food-rise-food-allergies-children>
54   'Food anaphylaxis in the United Kingdom: analysis of
     national data, 1998-2018'. Conrado et al, *The BMJ*, 2021.
     See: <https://www.bmj.com/content/372/bmj.n733>
55   <https://www.legislation.gov.uk/eur/2011/1169/contents>
56   'Survey of allergen advisory labelling and allergen content
     of UK retail pre-packed processed foods', B. Hirst, RSSL,

2014. See: <https://www.food.gov.uk/sites/default/files/
media/document/survey-allergen-labelling-prepacked.pdf>

57 'May contain traces' – what do doctors advise parents
of food allergic children?', Turner et al, *Clinical &
Experimental Allergy*, 2013. See (p.1466): <https://
onlinelibrary.wiley.com/doi/epdf/10.1111/cea.12197>

58 'Dietary management of peanut and tree nut allergy: what
exactly should patients avoid?', Brough et al, *Clinical &
Experimental Allergy*, 2014. See: <https://onlinelibrary.wiley.
com/doi/pdf/10.1111/cea.12466>

59 'Dietary management of peanut and tree nut allergy: what
exactly should patients avoid?', Brough et al, *Clinical &
Experimental Allergy*, 2014. See: <https://onlinelibrary.wiley.
com/doi/pdf/10.1111/cea.12466>

60 'Keeping food allergic children safe in our schools – time
for urgent action', Turner et al, *Clinical & Experimental
Allergy*, 2020. See: <https://onlinelibrary.wiley.com/doi/
full/10.1111/cea.13567>

61 Anaphylaxis Campaign: Making Schools Safer Project
2021. See: <https://www.anaphylaxis.org.uk/campaigning/
making-schools-safer-project/>

62 Spare Pens in Schools: <https://www.sparepensinschools.
uk/for-schools/staff-training-and-school-policies/>

63 'Child and parental reports of bullying in a consecutive
sample of children with food allergy', Shemesh et al,
Paediatrics, 2013. See <https://pubmed.ncbi.nlm.nih.
gov/23266926/>

64 'Psychological services for food allergy: the unmet need for
patients and families in the United Kingdom', Knibb et al,
Clinical & Experimental Allergy. See: <https://onlinelibrary.
wiley.com/doi/abs/10.1111/cea.13488>

65 'Parental Anxiety and Posttraumatic Stress Symptoms
(PTSS) in Paediatric Food Allergy', Roberts et al, *Journal of
Paediatric Psychology*, 2021. See: <https://pubmed.ncbi.nlm.
nih.gov/33704484/>

66 'Parental Anxiety and Posttraumatic Stress Symptoms in Paediatric Food Allergy', Roberts et al, *Journal of Paediatric Psychology*, 2021. See: <https://academic.oup.com/jpepsy/advance-article-abstract/doi/10.1093/jpepsy/jsab012/6163077?redirectedFrom=fulltext>

67 'Understanding the challenges faced by adolescents and young adults with allergic conditions: A systematic review', Vazquez-Ortiz et al, *Allergy*, 2020. See: <https://pubmed.ncbi.nlm.nih.gov/32141620/>

68 'The psychosocial impact of food allergy and food hypersensitivity in children, adolescents and their families: a review', Cummings et al, *Allergy*, 2010. See: <https://onlinelibrary.wiley.com/doi/10.1111/j.1398-9995.2010.02342.x>

69 'EAACI Guidelines on the effective transition of adolescents and young adults with allergy and asthma', Roberts et al, *Allergy*, 2020. See: <https://onlinelibrary.wiley.com/doi/full/10.1111/all.14459>

70 'Basophil Activation Test Reduces Oral Food Challenges to Nuts and Sesame', Santos et al, *The Journal of Allergy & Clinical Immunology*, 2020. See: <https://www.sciencedirect.com/science/article/pii/S2213219820314033>

Index

Anagnostou, Dr Katherine, 30–1
anaphylactic shock, 24
Anaphylaxis Campaign charity,
    35, 51, 72, 155, 191, 200, 236,
    256
anaphylaxis/anaphylactic reaction,
    2, 22–3
    from airborne allergens, 26–7
    biphasic reactions, 37–8
    coping afterwards, 230–2
    and hives, 102
    hospital treatment, 37–8
    recognizing, 23–4, 25–6
    risks, 24–5
    treatments, 24, 29–33
animals, 177, 283
    hygiene hypothesis, 80
antibiotics, 83
antibodies
    Immunoglobulin E (IgE)
        antibodies, 2
    tests for, 49
antihistamines, 29
    for anaphylaxis, 24
    carrying, 220–1
    effect on skin prick tests, 50
    for hay fever, 281
anxiety, 222–4
    about allergic reactions, 58
    about dying from allergies, 219
    about new food, 234–5
    about oral food challenges, 62–3
    about skin prick tests, 53–6
    after an anaphylactic reaction,
        230–2
    causes, 226–7
    discussing with your child,
        227–8
    gradual exposure ladder, 228–30
    management, 237–9
    modelling calm behaviour,
        232–3
    of parents, 64–7, 231
    resources for finding help, 236–7

seeking help for, 224–5
seeking reassurance, 235–6
self-help techniques, 231–2
signs of, 226–7
apples, Oral Allergy Syndrome
    (OAS), 5
apps, 117, 236–7
apricots, Oral Allergy Syndrome
    (OAS), 5
aquafaba, 165–6
asthma
    diagnosis of, 278–9
    symptoms, 278
    treatments, 279–80
atopic march, 71
atopy, 4, 47, 85, 86
Australia, 120
Auvi-Q device, 36–7
avocado, 20
    Latex Food Syndrome, 6

babies
    type of milk, 9–10, 88
    see also infants
Baby Biome study (2019), 82
bags for medication, 220–1, 260
bake sales, 150–2
baking
    in schools, 175
    see also recipes
bananas, 20, 286
    Latex Food Syndrome, 6
    outgrowing allergies, 70
barley, coeliac disease, 7
Basophil Activation Test (BAT),
    295
bathing, 276
beansprouts, Oral Allergy
    Syndrome (OAS), 5
bee stings, anaphylaxis/
    anaphylactic reaction, 22
Benadryl, 29
biome depletion, 81–2